Second Edition

Medicinal Chemistry II

Course Code **BP 501T**

for **Fifth Semester Bachelor in Pharmacy**

As per the latest syllabus prescribed by Pharmacy Council of India

Second Edition

Medicinal Chemistry II

Course Code **BP 501T**

for **FIFth Semester Bachelor in Pharmacy**

As per the latest syllabus prescribed by Pharmacy Council of India

K Ilango MPharm PhD FIC
Professor and Principal
Tagore College of Pharmacy
Chennai – 600 127

P Valentina MPharm PhD
Professor and Principal
PERI College of Pharmacy
Chennai – 600 048

CBSPD

CBS Publishers & Distributors Pvt Ltd

New Delhi • Bengaluru • Chennai • Kochi • Kolkata • Lucknow • Mumbai
Hyderabad • Jharkhand • Nagpur • Patna • Pune • Uttarakhand

Second Edition

Medicinal Chemistry II

Course Code **BP 501T**

for **Fifth Semester Bachelor in Pharmacy**

As per the latest syllabus prescribed by Pharmacy Council of India

ISBN: 978-93-49057-17-3

Second Edition: 2025
First Edition: 2019

Published by Satish Kumar Jain and produced by Varun Jain for
CBS Publishers and Distributors Pvt Ltd
4819/XI Prahlad Street, 24 Ansari Road, Daryaganj, New Delhi 110 002, India.
Ph: 011-23289259, 23266838 Website: www.cbspd.com
e-mail: delhi@cbspd.com

Corporate Office: 204 FIE, Industrial Area, Patparganj, Delhi 110 092, India
Ph: 011-49344934 Fax: 011-49344935 e-mail: publishing@cbspd.com; publicity@cbspd.com

Branches

- **Bengaluru:** Seema House 2975, 17th Cross, K.R. Road, Banasankari 2nd Stage, Bengaluru 560 070, Karnataka, India
  Ph: +91-80-26771678/79 Fax: +91-80-26771680 e-mail: bangalore@cbspd.com
- **Chennai:** 7, Subbarayan Street, Shenoy Nagar, Chennai 600 030, Tamil Nadu, India
  Ph: +91-44-42032115, 26681266 e-mail: chennai@cbspd.com
- **Kochi:** 42/1325, 1326, Power House Road, Opposite KSEB, Power House, Ernakulam 682 018, Kochi, Kerala, India
  Ph: +91-484-4059061–65 Fax: +91-484-4059065 e-mail: kochi@cbspd.com
- **Kolkata:** 147 Hind Ceramics Compound, 1st Floor, Nilgunj Road, Belghoria, Kolkata 700 056, West Bengal, India
  Ph: +91-33-25633055/56 e-mail: kolkata@cbspd.com
- **Lucknow:** Basement, Khushnuma Complex, 7-Meerabai Marg (Behind Jawahar Bhawan), Lucknow 226 001, Uttar Pradesh, India
  Ph: +91-522-4000032 e-mail:tiwari.lucknow@cbspd.com
- **Mumbai:** PWD Shed, Gala No. 25/26, Ramchandra Bhatt Marg, Next to JJ Hospital, Gate No. 2, Opp Union Bank of India, Noorbaug, Mumbai 400009, Maharashtra, India
  Ph: +91-22-66661880, 66661889 e-mail: mumbai@cbspd.com

Representatives

• **Hyderabad**	0-9885175004	• **Jharkhand**	0-9811541605	• **Nagpur**	0-8692091830
• **Patna**	0-9334159340	• **Pune**	0-9664372571	• **Uttarakhand**	0-9716462459

Printed at: SRK Graphics, Delhi, India

Preface

Medicinal chemistry is a vital discipline in drug discovery and development (DDD), bridging various scientific fields such as biology, toxicology, pharmacology, and more. This book, *Medicinal Chemistry II*, is the result of over 30 years of teaching and collaboration with graduate students across multiple universities. The positive feedback on our previous works, including *Textbook of Medicinal Chemistry*, Volumes I & II and *Medicinal Chemistry for Pharm D*, has inspired us to create this comprehensive yet accessible resource.

Designed for undergraduate students preparing for medicinal chemistry, this volume aligns with the revised syllabus of the Pharmacy Council of India. It consists of 13 chapters covering topics such as Antihistamines, Anticancer agents and Diuretics among others. Each chapter includes an introduction, classification, structure activity relationship (SAR), drug structures, IUPAC names, mechanisms of action, uses and synthesis all aimed at enhancing student understanding.

We extend our heartfelt thanks to our families and friends for their unwavering support, and we appreciate the faculty and students for their enthusiasm regarding our previous editions. We welcome suggestions for improvement and look forward to ongoing engagement with the academic community.

K Ilango
P Valentina

Contents

Preface *v*

Syllabus *xiii*

1. Antihistamines **1–27**

1. Introduction 1
   - 1.1 Histamine 1
   - 1.2 Biosynthesis of Histamine 1
   - 1.3 Chemistry of Histamine 2
   - 1.4 Histamine Receptors 3
2. Histamine Release Inhibitors - Mast Cell Stabilizers 4
3. Released Histamine Inhibitors 5
   - 3.1 Introduction 5
   - 3.2 Mechanism of action of Antihistamines 5
   - 3.3 Structure Activity Relationship 6
   - 3.4 Therapeutic Applications of Antihistamines 7
   - 3.5 Classification 8
     - 3.5.1 First Generation H_1 Antagonists 8
     - 3.5.2 Second Generation Antihistamines 20
     - 3.5.3 H_2-Receptor Antagonist 23
     - 3.5.4 Gastric Proton Pump Inhibitors 26

2. Antineoplastic Agents **28–49**

1. Introduction 28
2. Classification 29
   - 2.1 Alkylating Agents 30
   - 2.2 Antimetabolites 35
   - 2.3 Antibiotics 43
   - 2.4 Plant Products 46
   - 2.5 Hormones 48
   - 2.6 Miscellaneous 49

3. Antianginal Agents **50–60**

1. Introduction 50

2. Classification	50
2.1 Nitrite and Nitrates	51
2.2 Calcium Channel Blockers	53
2.2.1 1, 4 - Dihydro pyridine	54
2.2.2 Phenyl Alkylamine	57
2.2.3 Benzothiazepine	58
2.2.4 Diamino Propanol Ethers	59
2.3 Miscellaneous	59
4. Diuretics	**61–74**
1. Introduction	61
1.1 Mechanism of Action of Diuretics	61
1.2 Therapeutic Uses of Diuretics	62
2. Classification	62
2.1 *Carbonic Anhydrase* Inhibitors	63
2.2 Thiazide/Thiazide like Diuretics	66
2.3 High Ceiling or Loop Diuretics	69
2.4 Potassium Sparing Diuretics	71
2.5 Osmotic Diuretics	73
5. Antihypertensive Agents	**75–90**
1. Introduction	75
2. Classification	76
2.1 Adreno Receptor Antagonist	77
2.2 Adrenergic Neuron Blockers	78
2.3 Centrally Acting Agents	80
2.4 Vasodilators	82
2.5 Targeting Renin-Angiotensin System	86
6. Antiarrhythmic Agents	**91–98**
1. Introduction	91
2. Classification	91
2.1 Membrane Stabilizing Agents	92
2.2 β - Adrenergic Blocking Agents	97
2.3 Repolarization Prolongators	98
7. Antihyperlipidemic Agents	**99–104**
1. Introduction	99
2. Classification	100
2.1 *HMG - CoA Reductase* Inhibitors	101

2.2 Fibric acid Derivatives 102
2.3 Bile acid Sequestrants 103

8. Coagulants and Anticoagulants 105–110
1. Coagulants 105
2. Classification 105
3. Anticoagulants 107
3.1 Introduction 107
3.2 Mechanism of Action 107
3.3 Classification 108

9. Drugs for Congestive Heart Failure 111–121
1. Introduction 111
2. Classification 113
2.1 Inotropic Drugs 113
2.1.1 Cardiac Glycosides 113
2.2 Vasodilators 119
2.2.1 Synthetic Brain Natriuretic Peptide 119
2.2.2 Competitive Inhibitor of Endothelin 120

10. Steroidal Hormones 122–147
1. Introduction 122
1.1 Structure and Stereochemistry 122
1.2 Nomenclature 124
1.3 Procedure for Naming a Steroid 126
1.4 Biosynthesis and Metabolism 129
1.5 Mechanism of Action 130
2. Sex Hormones 131
2.1 Androgens 131
2.1.1 Classification 132
2.1.1.1 Natural Androgens 132
2.1.1.2 Anabolic Steroids 133
2.2 Gestogens 134
2.2.1 Classification 134
2.2.1.1 Progesterone and its Derivatives 135
2.3 Oestrogens 135
2.3.1 Classification 136
2.3.1.1 Natural Oestrogens 136
2.3.1.2 Synthetic Oestrogens 137

3. Drugs for Erectile Dysfunction 138
3.1 Introduction 138
4. Oral Contraceptives 139
4.1 Introduction 139
4.2 Type of contraceptives 140
4.2.1 Steroidal contraceptives 140
5. Adrenal Cortical Hormones 143
5.1 Introduction 143
5.2 Glucocorticoids 144
5.2.1 Classification 144
5.2.1.1 Natural Glucocorticoids 145
5.2.1.2 Synthetic Glucocorticoids 146
5.2.1.3 Fluoro Derivatives 146

11. Thyroid and Antithyroid Drugs **148–153**
1. Thyroid Drugs 148
1.1 Introduction 148
1.2 Bio-synthesis of Thyroid Hormone 148
1.3 Thyroid Dysfunctions 150
1.4 Synthetic Thyroid Hormones 150
2. Antithyroid Drugs 152
2.1 Introduction 152
2.2 Classification 152
2.2.1 Thioamides 153

12. Antidiabetic Agents **154–166**
1. Introduction 154
2. Insulin 155
2.1 Introduction 155
2.2 Production of Insulin 156
2.3 Insulin Preparation 156
3. Oral Hypoglycemic Agents 160
3.1 Introduction 160
3.2 Classification 160
3.2.1 Sulfonyl Ureas 160
3.2.2 Biguanides 162
3.2.3 Thiazolidinones 163
3.2.4 Metaglinides 164
3.2.5 α-*Glucosidase* Inhibitors 165

13. Local Anaesthetics **167–182**

1. Introduction 167
    1.1 Mechanism of Action 167
    1.2 Structure Activity Relationship 168
2. Classification 170
    2.1 Ester Based 171
        2.1.1 Natural Agents 171
        2.1.2 Synthetic Agents 172
    2.2 Amide Based 178
    2.3 Miscellaneous 181

Index *183–185*

Syllabus

BP501T Medicinal Chemistry II (Theory)

Unit I **10 hrs**

(a) Antihistaminic Agents: Histamine, receptors and their distribution in the human body

H1-Antagonists: Diphenhydramine hydrochloride*, Dimenhydrinate, Doxylamine succinate, Clemastine fumarate, Diphenylpyraline hydrochloride, Tripelennamine hydrochloride, Chlorcyclizine hydrochloride, Meclizine hydrochloride, Buclizine hydrochloride, Chlorpheniramine maleate, Triprolidine hydrochloride*, Phenindamine tartrate, Promethazine hydrochloride*, Trimeprazine tartrate, Cyproheptadine hydrochloride, Azatadine maleate, Astemizole , Loratadine, Cetirizine, Levocetirizine, Cromolyn sodium.

H2-Antagonists: Cimetidine*, Famotidine, Ranitidine.

Gastric Proton Pump Inhibitors: Omeprazole, Lansoprazole, Pantoprazole, Rabeprazole.

(b) Antineoplastic Agents:

Alkylating Agents: Mechlorethamine*, Cyclophosphamide, Melphalan, Chlorambucil, Busulfan, Thiotepa,

Antimetabolites: Mercaptopurine*, Thioguanine, Fluorouracil, Floxuridine, Cytarabine, Methotrexate*, Azathioprine.

Antibiotics: Dactinomycin, Daunorubicin, Doxorubicin, Bleomycin.

Plant Products: Etoposide, Vinblastine sulphate, Vincristine sulphate.

Miscellaneous: Cisplatin, Mitotane.

Unit II **10 hrs**

(a) Antianginal Agents:
Vasodilators: Amyl nitrate, Nitroglycerin*, Pentaerythritol tetranitrate, Isosorbide dinitrate*, Dipyridamole.

Calcium Channel Blockers: Verapamil, Bepridil hydrochloride, Diltiazem hydrochloride, Nifedipine, Amlodipine, Felodipine, Nicardipine, Nimodipine.

(b) Diuretics:
***Carbonic anhydrase* Inhibitors:** Acetazolamide*, Methazolamide, Dichlorphenamide.

Thiazides: Chlorthiazide*, Hydrochlorthiazide, Hydroflumethiazide, Cyclothiazide.

Loop Diuretics: Furosemide, Bumetanide, Ethacrynic acid.

Potassium Sparing Diuretics: Spironolactone, Triamterene, Amiloride.

Osmatic Diuretics: Mannitol

(c) Antihypertensive Agents: Timolol, Captopril, Lisinopril, Enalapril, Benazepril hydrochloride, Quinapril hydrochloride, Methyldopate hydrochloride*, Clonidine hydrochloride, Guanethidine monosulphate, Guanabenz acetate, Sodium nitroprusside, Diazoxide, Minoxidil, Reserpine, Hydralazine hydrochloride.

Unit III **10 hrs**

(a) Antiarrhythmic Agents: Quinidine sulphate, Procainamide hydrochloride, Disopyramide phosphate*, Phenytoin sodium, Lidocaine hydrochloride, Tocaine hydrochloride, Mexiletine hydrochloride, Lorcainide hydrochloride, Amiodarone, Sotalol.

(b) Antihyperlipidemic Agents: Clofibrate, Lovastatin, Cholesteramine and Cholestipol.

(c) Coagulants and Anticoagulants: Meandione, Acetomenaphthone, Warfarin*, Anisindione, Clopidogrel.

(d) Drugs used in Congestive Heart Failure: Digoxin, Digitoxin, Nesiritide, Bosentan, Tezosentan.

Unit IV **08 hrs**

Drugs acting on Endocrine System: Nomenclature and metabolism of steroids.

Sex hormones: Testosterone, Nandrolone, Progesterone, Oestriol, Oestradiol, Oestrione, Diethylstilbestrol.

Drugs for Erectile Dysfunction: Sildenafil, Tadalafil.

Oral Contraceptives: Mifepristone, Norgestril, Levonorgestrol.

Corticosteroids: Cortisone, Hydrocortisone, Prednisolone, Betamethasone, Dexamethasone.

Thyroid and Antithyroid Drugs: L-Thyroxine, L-Thyronine, Propyl thiouracil, Methimazole.

Unit V **07 hrs**

(a) Antidiabetic Agents: Insulin and its preparation

Sulfonyl Ureas: Tolbutamide*, Chlorpropamide, Glipizide, Glimepiride.

Biguanides: Metformin

Thiazolidinediones: Pioglitazone, Rosiglitazone.

Meglitinides: Repaglinide, Nateglinide.

Glucosidase Inhibitors: Acarbose, Voglibose.

(b) Local Anesthetics: SAR of Local anesthetics

Benzoic Acid Derivatives: Cocaine, Hexylcaine, Meprylcaine, Cyclomethycaine, Piperocaine.

Amino Benzoic Acid Derivatives: Benzocaine*, Butamben, Procaine*, Butacaine, Propoxycaine, Tetracaine, Benoxinate.

Lidocaine/Anilide Derivatives: Lignocaine, Mepivacaine, Prilocaine, Etidocaine.

Miscellaneous: Phenacaine, Diperadon, Dibucaine*.

ANTIHISTAMINES

Chapter
1

1. INTRODUCTION

The term antihistamine implies to drug that reduces or eliminates the effects mediated by the chemical histamine. The term antihistamine refers only to H_1 receptor antagonist.

1.1 Histamine

Histamine is a neurotransmitter or chemical messenger that carries signals from one nerve to another, as well as performing several other important functions in various bodily tissues. Histamine is an autacoid, which means it acts similarly to a local hormone, near its site of synthesis. It is a β-imidazolyl ethylamine derivative, distributed in mast cells in all peripheral tissues of the body and basophils in the blood. It is produced naturally by immune system and released in response to tissue damage. It mediates immediate allergic and inflammatory response, causes gastric acid release and function as a central nervous system neurotransmitter. Systemically, histamine contracts smooth muscle of lungs and gastrointestinal system and cause vasodilatation, low blood pressure and increases heart rate. It causes symptoms such as itching, sneezing, watery eye and runny nose.

1.2 Biosynthesis of Histamine

In the living organism, histamine is synthesized from the naturally occurring α-amino acid, histidine by the loss of a carboxyl group through bacteria or enzymatic decarboxylation. It is synthesized in the Golgi apparatus of mast cells and basophils. This conversion is catalyzed by *L-histidine decarboxylase*.

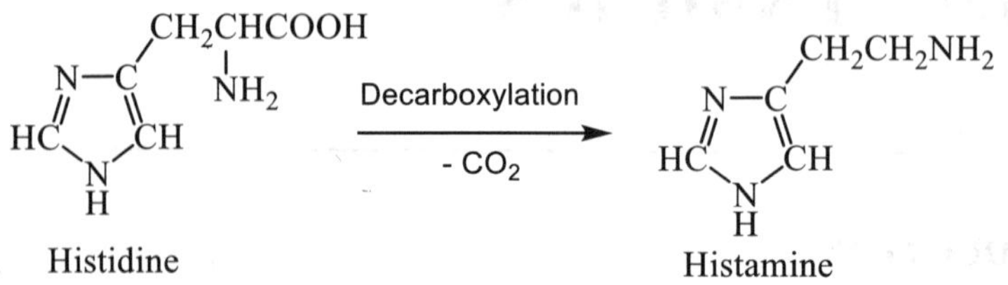

1.3 Chemistry of Histamine

Histamine is 4 - (2- Amino ethyl) imidazole, structurally composed of an imidazole and ethyl amine side chain. The methylene group of amino ethyl side chain is designated as α and β. The side chain attached via β-CH_2 to the 4th position of imidazole ring. The nitrogen at position 3 is designated as pros (π) and 1 is termed as (τ) tele.

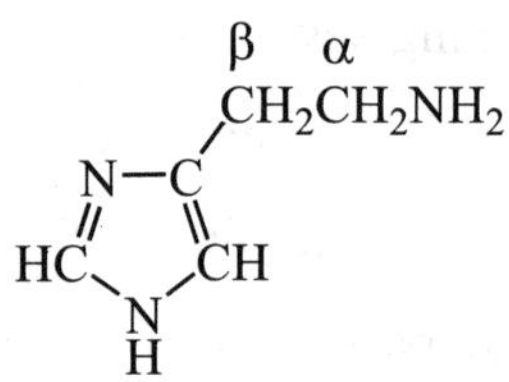

Histamine

At physiological pH, the amino nitrogen atom at the side chain is protonated. Histamine occurs therefore, as a monovalent cation, which forms an intramolecular hydrogen bond between side chain amino nitrogen and ring nitrogen.

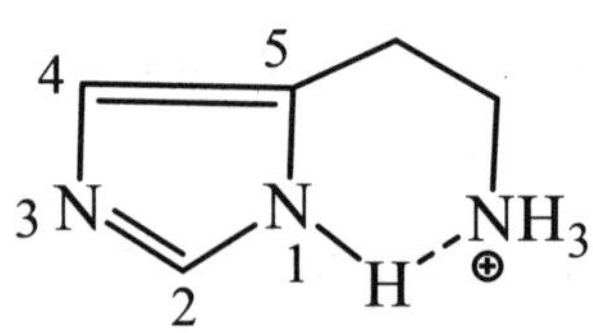

Histamine is an achiral molecule, histamine receptors are stereo selective toward chiral ligand. Studies with conformational restricted histamine analogues suggest that *trans* rotamer possess affinity for both H_1 and H_2 histamine receptors, the Gauche conformer act at H_3 receptors

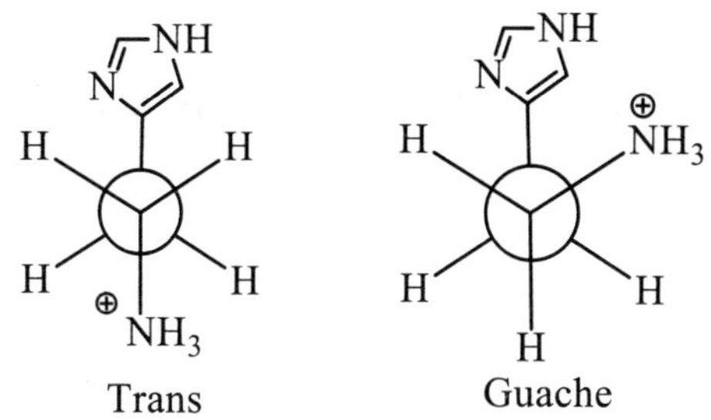

Histamine rotamers

1.4 Histamine Receptors

Histamine receptors belong to the G-protein coupled receptor family. These receptors are divided into four subtypes H_1, H_2, H_3 and H_4 according to their function, structure, distribution and their affinity to histamine.

i) H_1 receptors

It is found in smooth muscles of intestine, bronchi, blood vessels, adrenal medulla, endothelial cell and lymphocytes. The H_1-receptor protein is G-protein coupled, linked to intercellular Gq, which activates *phospholipase C* and increases intracellular Ca^{++} levels. All immediate hypersensitivity reactions, including symptoms observed in the skin, such as erythema, pruritus edema, broncho-constriction, motion sickness, smooth muscle relaxation and vasodilation may be due to activation of H_1 receptor. Antagonist of H_1 receptor are used as antiallergic and antiemetics.

ii) H_2 receptor

It is present in the tissues of parietal cells located in the stomach lining, myocardial cell, uterus and vascular smooth muscle cells. Histamine action at these receptors, stimulates the release of gastric acid, inhibit antibody and cytokine production. H_2antagonists are used as antiulcer.

iii) H_3 receptor

It is presynaptic receptor inhibit the synthesis and release of histamine in the histaminergic neurons in the central nervous system (CNS).

iv) H_4 receptor

The H_4 receptors found on immune cells and tissues including peripheral blood leukocytes, spleen, small intestine, bone marrow and thymus. Histamine action on these receptors, regulate the levels of white blood cell release from bone marrow. They have also been showing to direct mast cells.

Histamine antagonists are drugs that inhibit the effects of histamine by blocking or binding to H receptors. Histamine inhibitors are classified into

(A) **Histamine release inhibitors**

(B) **Released histamine inhibitors**

(i) H_1 antagonist- antihistamines (ii) H_2 antagonist - antiulcer

2. HISTAMINE RELEASE INHIBITORS - MAST CELL STABILIZERS

These agents stabilize mast cell and inhibit the release of histamine and other mediators of inflammation. Generally, the mast cell stabilizer inhibit activation and mediator release from a variety of inflammatory cell type associated with allergy and asthma, including eosinophils, neutrophils, macrophages, mast cell, monocytes and platelets.

A. Cromolyn sodium (Crolom)

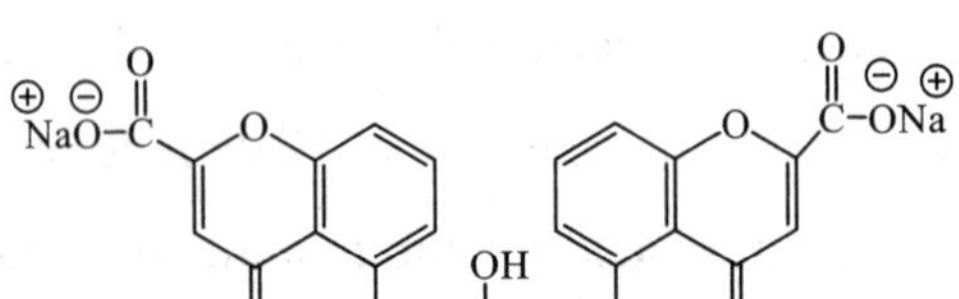

Disodium - 1, 3 - bis - (2 - carboxychromon - 5 - yloxy) - 2 - hydroxy propane

Mechanism of action: It stabilizes mast cell and inhibits the release of histamine and anaphylaxis (SRS-A), a Type I allergic reaction. It may also reduce the release of inflammatory leukotrienes.

Use: It is used for bronchial asthma for prevention of induced bronchospasm and rhinitis (nasal solution). Topically used as eye drops for allergic conjunctivitis and keratitis.

3. RELEASED HISTAMINE INHIBITORS

(H_1 ANTAGONIST-ANTIHISTAMINES)

3.1 Introduction

Antihistamines are the drugs that inhibit the release of histamines at H_1 receptor. The first generation H_1 antihistamines are useful in the treatment of allergic response like hay fever, rhinitis, urticaria and food allergy. H_2 antagonists interact with H_2 receptors and primarily used in the treatment of peptic ulcer and other gastric hyper secretory states.

First-generation H_1 antihistamines readily cross the blood-brain barrier (BBB) and occupy H_1-receptors located on postsynaptic membranes of histaminergic neurons throughout the CNS. So, these agents act on adrenergic, cholinergic, dopaminergic and serotonergic receptor. This results in adverse effects like sedation, drowsiness, blurred vision, dry mouth, urinary retention, appetite stimulation, muscle spasm and CNS depression. This was overcome in second generation antihistamines, which do not cross the BBB and has less anticholinergic and CNS effect.

3.2 Mechanism of action of Antihistamines

The antihistamines have been used extensively for the symptomatic treatment (sneezing, rhinorrhea and itching of eyes, nose, and throat) of allergic rhinitis, chronic idiopathic urticaria and a number of other histamine related diseases. These uses are due to their antagonism action for histamine at peripheral H_1 receptors. The histamine (H_1)

receptors like other G-protein coupled receptors exist as equilibrium between the inactive state and the active state. Histamine stabilizes the receptor in its active conformation, thus causing the equilibrium to swing to the 'on' position. H_1 antihistamines act as inverse agonists that combine with and stabilize the inactive conformation of the H_1-receptor, shifting the equilibrium towards the inactive state and produce the opposite effect. It prevents the action of histamine mainly in immediate hypersensitivity. They act in the bronchi, capillaries and some other smooth muscles and are used to relieve motion sickness, seasonal rhinitis and allergic dermatitis.

A number of the antihistamines, particularly the phenothiazines and amino alkyl ethers, have antiemetic actions and thus useful in the treatment of nausea, vomiting and motion sickness.It blocks the histamine receptors in the vomiting center and affects the medullary chemoreceptor trigger zone. Certain antihistamines block central muscarinic receptors as a result they have limited use in Parkinson-like syndromes.

3.3 Structure Activity Relationship

The essential pharmacophore for H_1 antagonistic activity is represented by a general structure of 2 aromatic groups linked through a short chain to a tertiary aliphatic amine:

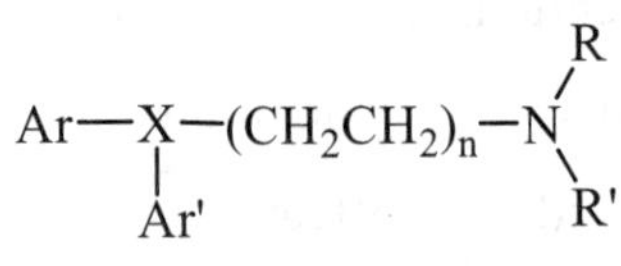

- ✓ The Ar group may be phenyl, substituted phenyl or hetero aryl group such as 2- pyridyl Ar' is a second aryl or aryl methyl group.
- ✓ X is a connecting atom of O, C or N; Chemical classification of these agents are usually based on the unit X which may be saturated Carbon-Oxygen (amino alkyl ether),

nitrogen (ethylene diamine) or carbon (propylamine) Tricyclic derivative in which two aromatic rings are bridged. eg. Phenothiazine.

- ✓ $(CH_2)_n$ is a carbon chain usually ethyl.
- ✓ NRR' represents basic terminal amine function. The diaryl substitution is essential for significant H_1 affinity.
- ✓ The nitrogen should be 3° amine in nature for maximum antihistaminic activity. The 'N' may also form a part of heterocyclic moieties like piperidine or piperazine. The nitrogen should be separated by 5-6 A° from the aromatic or hetero aromatic group.
- ✓ The group present between nitrogen atom and group X may be saturated or unsaturated or substituted.
- ✓ Many antihistamines contain a carbon atom in the connecting atom (X) are chiral and exhibit stereo selective receptor binding. eg. S-configuration of Pheniramine series has more affinity for H_1 receptor.

3.4 Therapeutic Applications of Antihistamines

Antihistamines are in general used in various

- ✓ allergic rhinitis (common cold),
- ✓ allergic conjunctivitis (pink eye),
- ✓ allergic dermatological conditions, urticaria (hives),
- ✓ angioedema (swelling of the skin),
- ✓ vertigo and Motion sickness,
- ✓ antiemetic and
- ✓ sedation (first generation H_1-antihistamines)

3.5 Classification

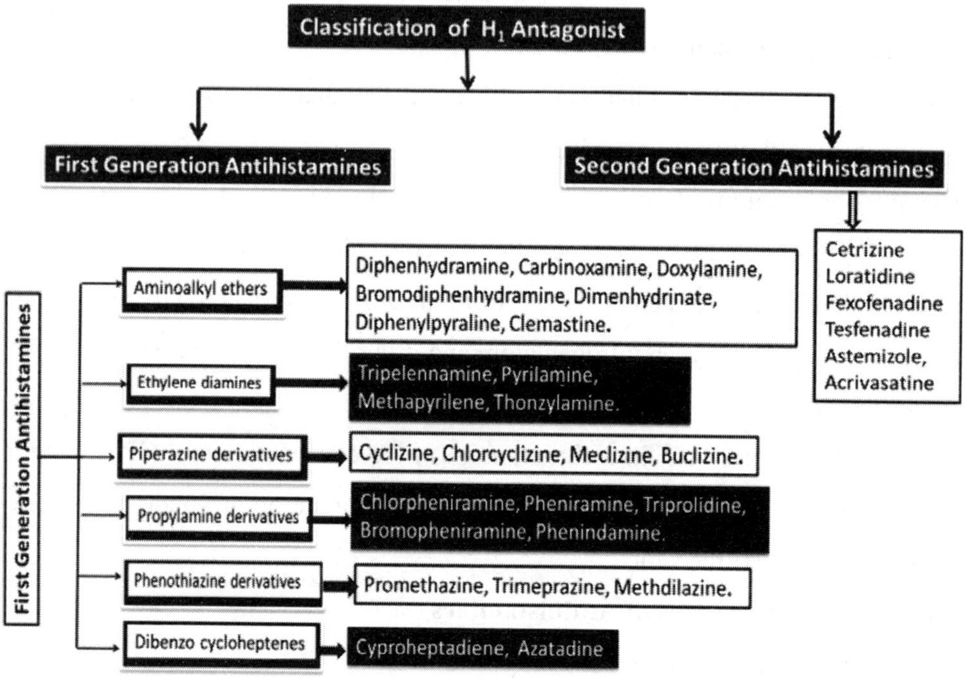

3.5.1 FIRST GENERATION H$_1$ ANTAGONISTS

3.5.1.1 Amino Alkyl Ethers

The best structure of amino-alkyl ethers 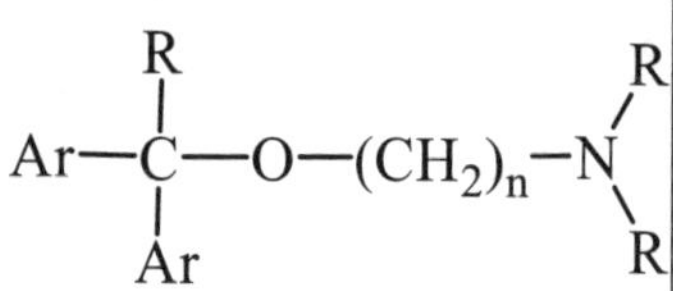	Ar group may be phenyl or substituted phenyl or heterocyclic for good antihistaminic activity
	The R group may be methyl or hydrogen
	If double bond is introduced between α, β-carbon atoms of the propyl chain drowsiness is produced
	In compounds with asymmetric carbon atom, the dextroisomer is more active

A. Diphenhydramine hydrochloride (Allerdryl)

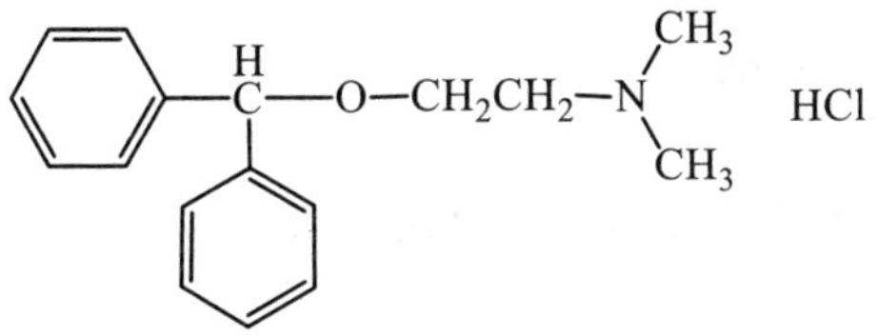

2 - (Diphenyl methoxy) - N, N' - dimethyl ethanamine hydrochloride

Synthesis

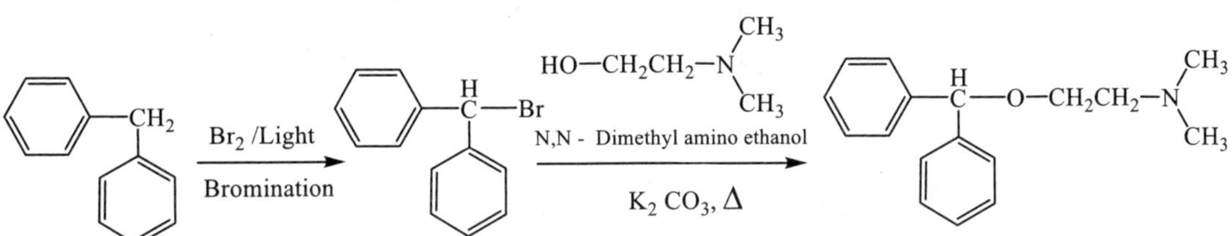

Diphenyl methane

Diphenhydramine

Mechanism of action: It acts as H_1 - receptor antagonist.

Use: In addition to antihistaminic activity, Diphenhydramine exhibits antiemetic, antitussive and sedative properties. It may be used as a nighttime sedative, for the control of drug induced Parkinsonism and in liquid form for control of cough.

B. Dimenhydrinate (Gravol)

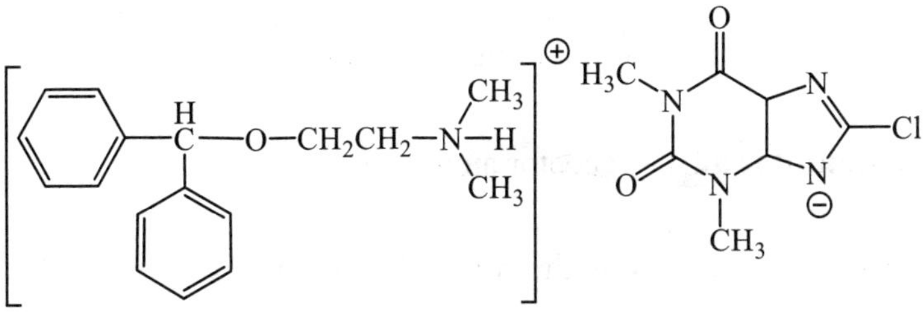

8 - Chloro - 3, 7 - dihydro - 1, 3 - dimethyl - 1H - purin - 2, 6 - dione compound with - 2 - (Diphenyl - N, N - dimethyl ethyl amine

Dimenhydrinate is 8-Chloro theophylline salt of Diphenhydramine. The salt of 8-chloro theophylline is used to overcome the common side effect (drowsiness and nervousness) of Diphenhydramine.

Mechanism of action: It is a H_1 - receptor antagonist.

Use: It is widely used to treat pregnancy and motion sickness induced nausea.

C. Doxylamine succinate (Aldex AN)

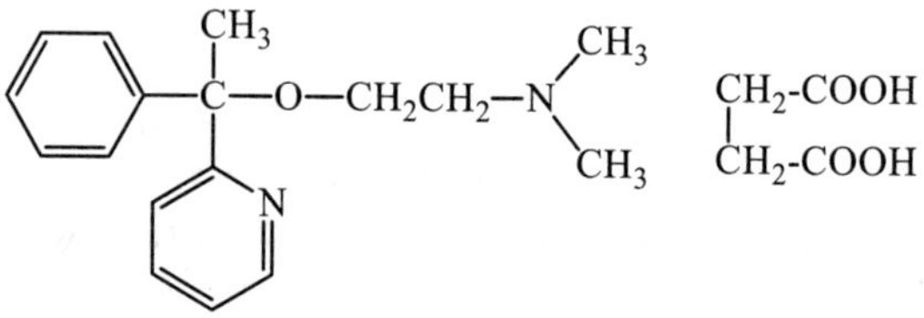

2 - [(1 - Phenyl) - 1 - (pyridin - 2 - yl) - ethoxy] - N, N - dimethyl ethanamine butanedioic acid

Mechanism of action: It is H_1 - receptor antagonist.

Use: It is an antihistaminic agent, but it has sedative property. It is also used with anti-tussive and decongestants for the relief of cough and cold.

D. Clemastine fumarate (Tavegyl)

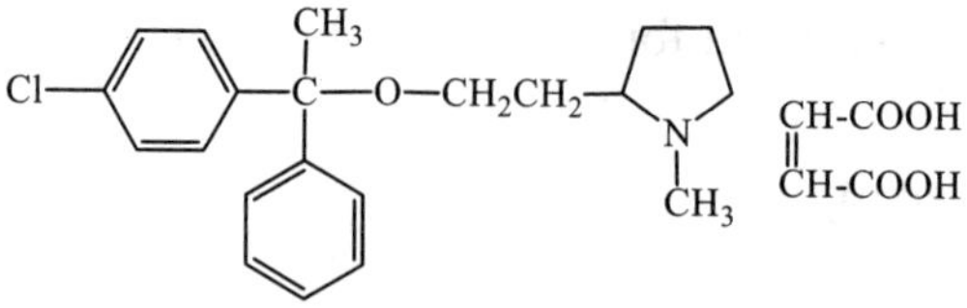

R - 2 - {2 - [1 - (p - Chloro phenyl) - 1 - phenyl ethoxy] ethyl} - 1 - methyl pyrrolidin but - 2 - enedioic acid

Mechanism of action: It is a H_1 – receptor antagonist.

Use: It has antihistaminic activity with anticholinergic and sedative effect. It is used for relief of allergic condition such as urticaria, rhinitis and conjunctivitis.

E. Diphenylpyraline hydrochloride (Corytab)

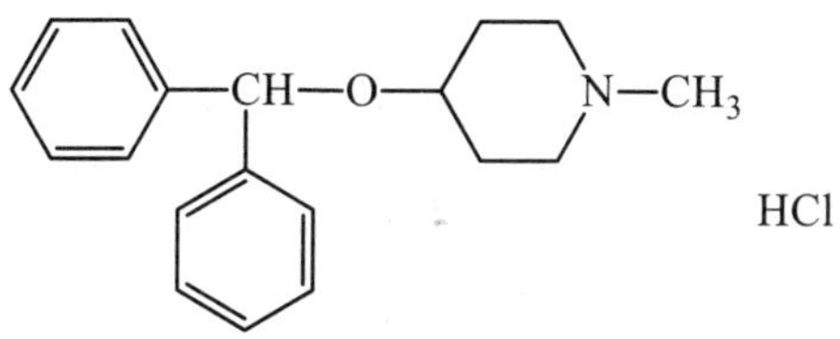

4 - (Diphenyl methoxy) -1- methyl
piperidine hydrochloride

Structurally it is related to Diphenhydramine with the amino alkyl side chain incorporated in a piperidine ring.

Mechanism of action: It is a H_1- receptor antagonist.

Use: It is a potent antihistaminic agent used in the treatment of allergic rhinitis, hay fever and allergic skin disorders.

3.5.1.2 Ethylenediamines

Basic structure of ethylenediamine derivatives of H_1antagonist 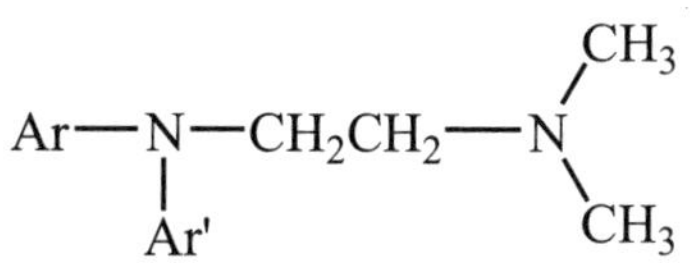	Ar' group by 2 - pyridinyl system yield more significant antihistamine. Substitution by p-methoxy further enhances activity
	All the compounds of this series have two 3° nitrogen which are separated by a two-carbon chain
	Terminal amino group is required for H_1 blocking activity
	They are highly effective H_1 antagonist and are useful antihistamine. They also exhibit high frequency CNS depression and gastrointestinal effects.

A. Tripelennamine hydrochloride (Pyribenzamine)

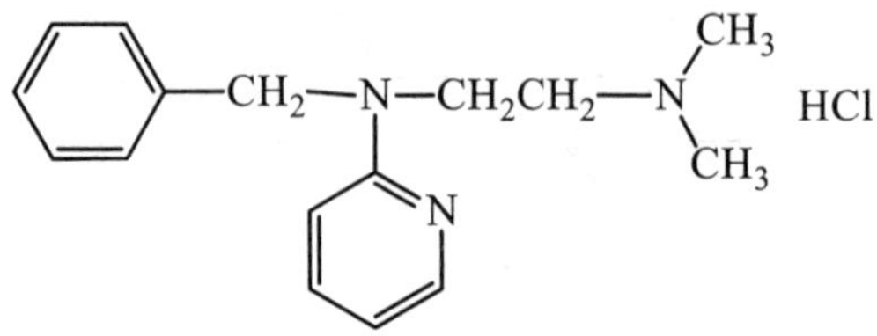

2 - {Benzyl [2 - (dimethyl amino) ethyl] amino}
pyridine hydrochloride

Mechanism of action: It is a H_1- receptor antagonist.

Use: It is used in the treatment of hay fever, urticaria and other mild allergic conditions.

3.5.1.3 Piperazine Derivatives

Piperazine derivatives are moderately potent antihistaminic with a lower incident of drowsiness. These agents are used to treat motion sickness and vertigo. The general structure of piperazine derivatives with some examples are given in Table 1.2

Table 1.2 Piperazine Derivatives

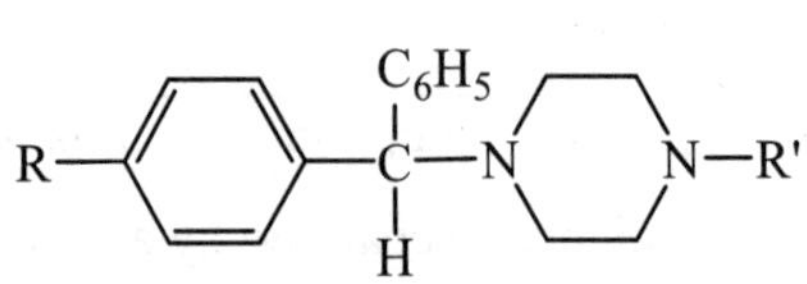		
Name	**R**	**R'**
Chlorcyclizine	- Cl	- CH_3
Meclizine	- Cl	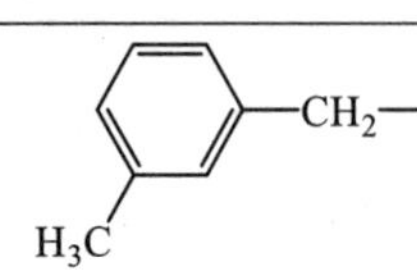 3 - Methyl benzyl

Buclizine	- Cl	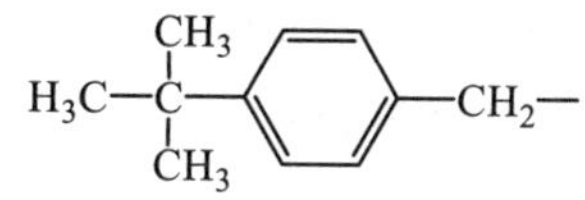 4 - t - Butyl benzyl

A. Chlorcyclizine hydrochloride (Ahist)

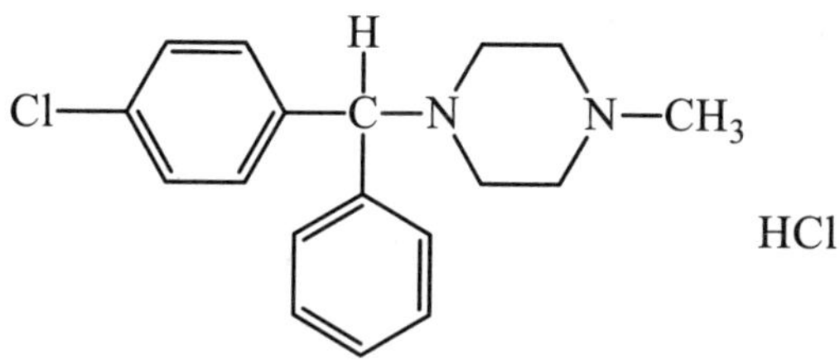

1 - [(4 - Chlorophenyl) phenyl methyl]- 4 - methyl piperazine hydrochloride

Mechanism of action: It acts as antihistamine by inhibiting the histamine at H_1 receptors. Chlorcyclizine also has some local anesthetic, anticholinergic and antiserotonergic properties and can be used as an antiemetic. It blocks the histamine receptors in the vomiting centre and affect the medullary chemoreceptor trigger zone.

Use: It is used in relief of urticaria, hay fever and certain other allergic conditions. It is also used as an antiemetic.

B. Meclizine hydrochloride (Antivert)

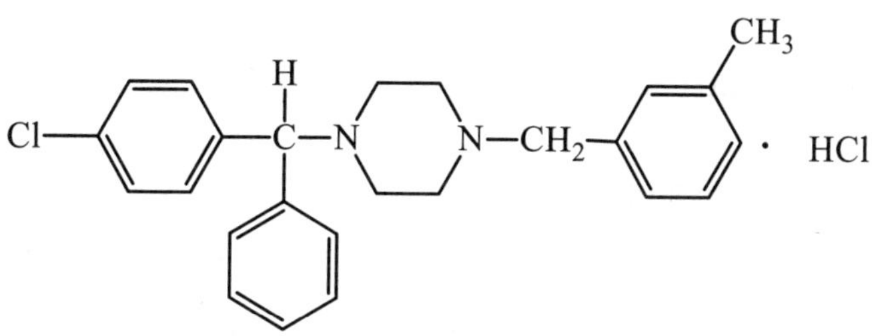

1- [(4 - Chloro phenyl) phenyl methyl] - 4 - (3 - methyl benzyl) piperazine hydrochloride

Mechanism of action: It acts as antihistamine by inhibiting the histamine at H_1 receptors. It blocks the histamine receptors in the vomiting center and affects the medullary chemoreceptor trigger zone.

Use: It is a moderate antihistamine. It is used to treat nausea and vomiting.

C. Buclizine hydrochloride (Longifene)

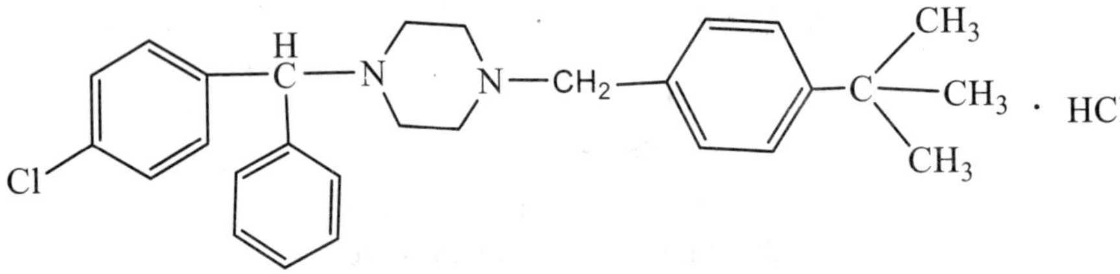

1- [(4 - t -Butyl phenyl) methyl] - 4 - [(4 - chloro phenyl) (phenyl) methyl] piperazine hydrochloride

Mechanism of action: It is an antihistamine with anti-muscarinic and moderate sedative properties. It is used mainly for its antiemetic activity. It is a potent H_1 receptor antihistaminic agent. It blocks the histamine receptors in the vomiting centre and thus affects the medullary chemoreceptor trigger zone. Furthermore, since Buclizine possesses anti-cholinergic properties as well, the muscarinic receptors are similarly blocked.

Use: It is used as an anti-vertigo and antiemetic agent.

3.5.1.4 Propylamine Derivatives

General structure of propylamine derivatives is

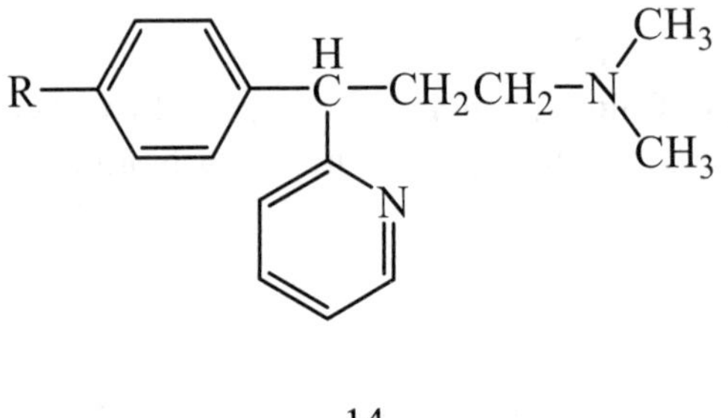

Propylamine derivatives contains an asymmetric carbon atom, the *dextro* rotatory isomer exhibit the greater potency. Introduction of chloro or bromo group in the benzene ring of Pheniramine increases its potency with no appreciable change in toxicity

Propylamine with connecting moiety include simple open chain alkene or cyclic alkene eg. Triprolidine, Phenindamine. In open chain double bond system appears to be an important factor for antihistaminic property. These compounds are asymmetric; E-isomer is more predominant than Z-isomer. The saturated member of this series are called Pheniramine. These agents produce less sedation than other classical antihistamines.

A. Chlorpheniramine maleate (Cadistin)

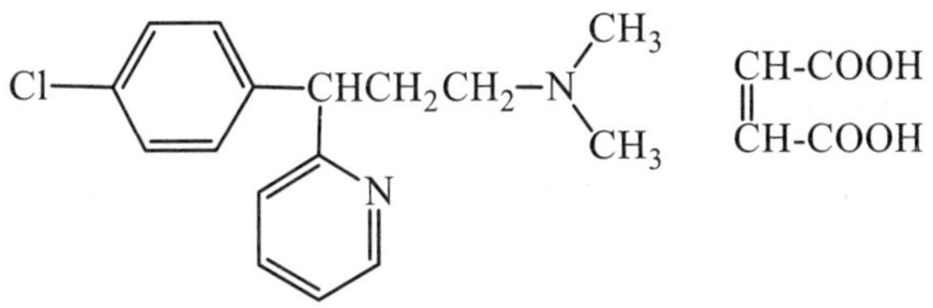

RS - 3 - (4 - Chloro phenyl) - 3 - (2 - pyridinyl) propyl dimethyl amine - but - 2 - enedioic acid

Mechanism of action: It competes with histamine for H_1 receptor sites on effectors cells in the gastrointestinal (GI) tract, blood vessels and respiratory tract. It provides effective temporary relief of sneezing, watery and itchy eyes and runny nose due to hay fever and other upper respiratory allergies.

Use: It is used in symptomatic relief of hyper sensitive reaction like urticaria, rhinitis, conjunctivitis and angioedema.

B. Triprolidine hydrochloride (Histex)

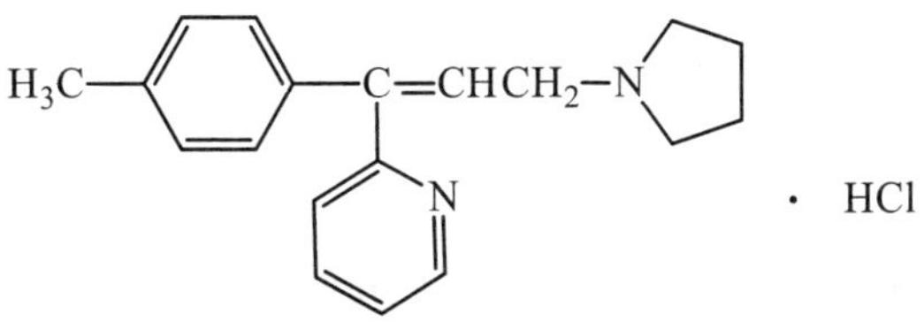

E - 2 - [3 - (Pyrrolidin - 1- yl) - 1 - (4 - tolyl) propenyl] pyridine hydrochloride

Synthesis

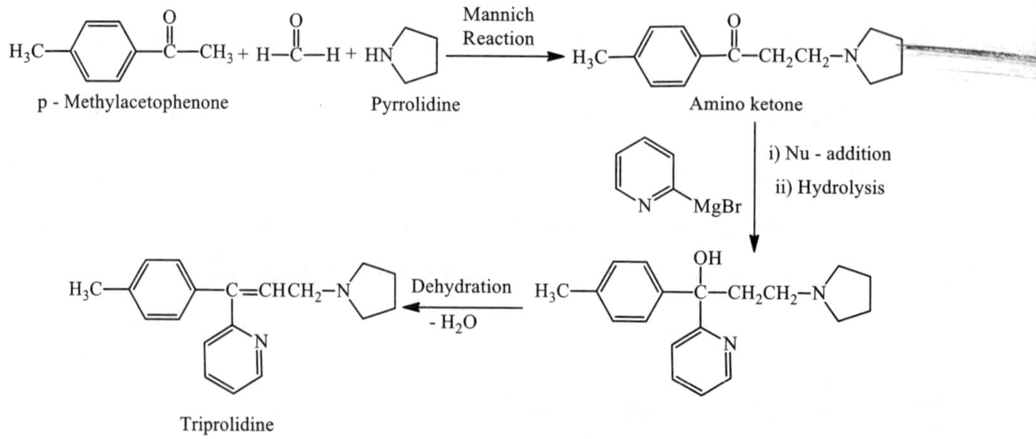

Mechanism of action: They compete with histamine for H_1-receptor sites on effector cells in the gastrointestinal (GI) tract, blood vessels, and respiratory tract.

Use: It is a potent antihistamine used for the relief of hypersensitivity including urticaria, rhinitis, conjunctivitis and skin disorders. It is used with Pseudo ephedrine for the treatment of cough and common cold.

C. Phenindamine tartrate (Nolahist)

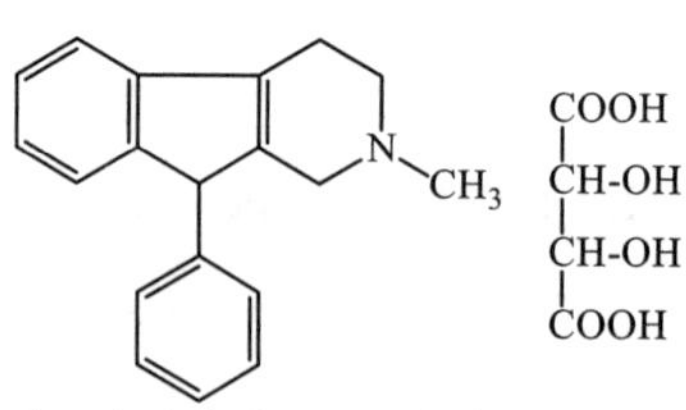

2 - Methyl - 9 - phenyl - 1, 3, 4, 9 - tetrahydro indeno [[2,1-c] - pyridine - 2, 3 - dihydroxy butanedioic acid

Mechanism of action: They compete with histamine for H_1- receptor sites and antagonize the effect of histamine.

Use: It is used in the treatment of common cold and allergies such as sneezing, itching and rashes.

3.5.1.5 Phenothiazine Derivatives

Phenothiazines possess tricyclic system. Phenothiazine derivatives possess two or three carbon chain bridge between basic phenothiazine nucleus and basic nitrogen. This differs from the phenothiazine antipsychotic series in which unbranched propyl chain is required. The phenothiazine ring is formed by treating the corresponding diphenylamine with a mixture of iodine and sulphur.

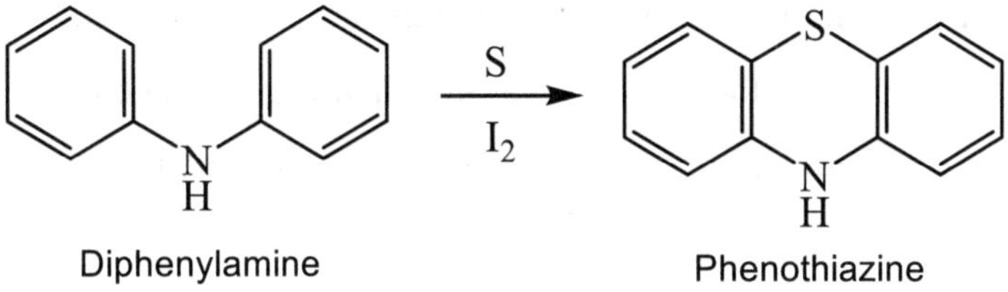

The proton on the nitrogen is weakly acidic, so a strong bases are required to form an anion in order to carry out the subsequent alkylation. Phenothiazine containing 2 or 3 carbon branched alkyl group between the ring and terminal nitrogen possess antihistaminic property. These derivatives with unbranched propyl chain exhibit antipsychotic activity.

A. Promethazine hydrochloride (Phenergan)

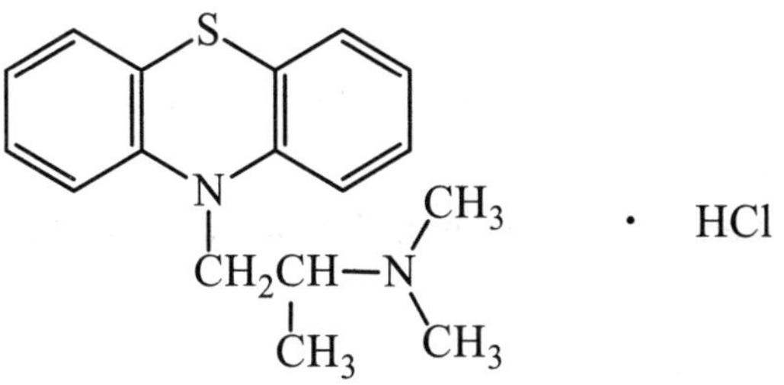

10 - [2 - (Dimethyl amino) propyl] phenothiazine hydrochloride

Synthesis

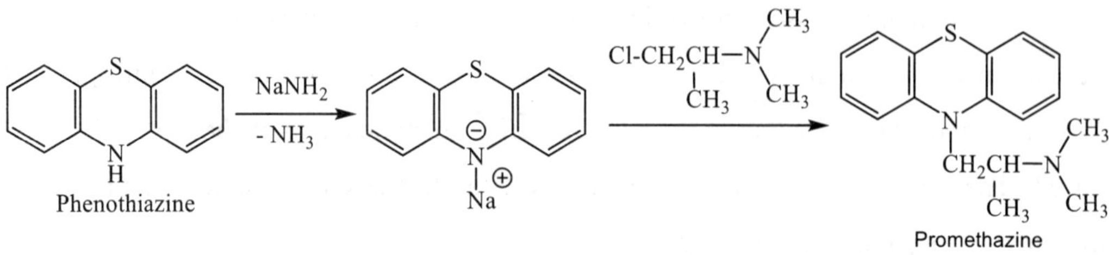

Mechanism of action: It competes with free histamine for binding at H_1 receptor sites in the GI tract, uterus, large blood vessel and bronchial muscle. The relief of nausea appears to be related to central anticholinergic actions and on the medullary chemoreceptor trigger zone.

Use: It is used as antihistaminic, antiemetic, tranquillizer, analgesic and sedative.

B. Trimeprazine tartrate (Alimemazine)

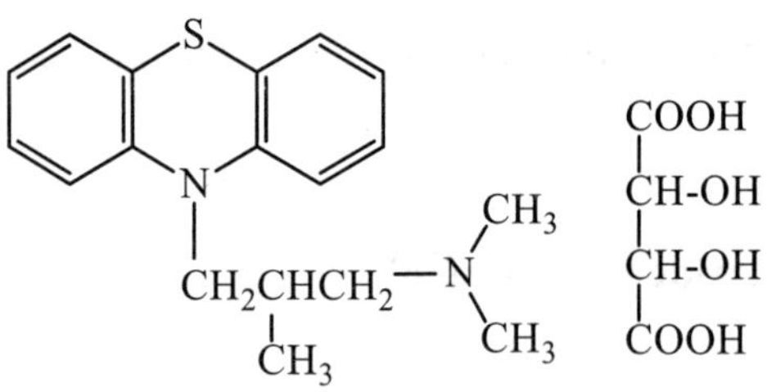

10 - [2 - (Dimethyl amino) propyl] phenothiazine - 2, 3 - dihydroxy butanedioic acid

Mechanism of action: It acts as antihistamine by inhibiting the histamine at H_1 receptors

Use: It is mainly used as antipruritic.

3.5.1.6 Dibenzo Cycloheptene Derivatives

A. Cyproheptadine hydrochloride (Apeplus)

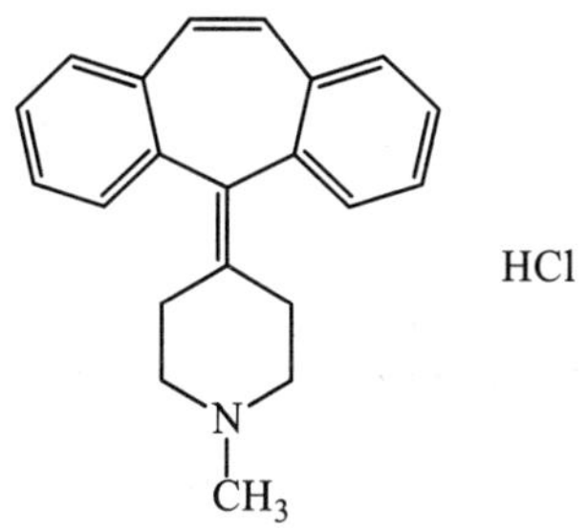

4 - (5H) - Dibenzo - [a, d] - cyclohepten - 5 - ylidene) - 1- methyl piperidine hydrochloride

Mechanism of action: It is a H_1-antagonists, act by competing with histamine for H_1-receptor sites on effector cells. It also has potent 5-HT (serotonin) antagonist activity through its 5-HT_{2A} receptor-blocking action. Antagonism of serotonin on the appetite center of the hypothalamus may account for its ability to stimulate appetite. In addition, it also has weak anticholinergic and central depressant properties.

Use: It possess both antihistaminic and anti-serotonin properties. It is also used as antipruritic agent, appetite stimulant, antiallergic and for the post gastrectomy dumping syndrome.

B. Azatadine maleate (Zadine)

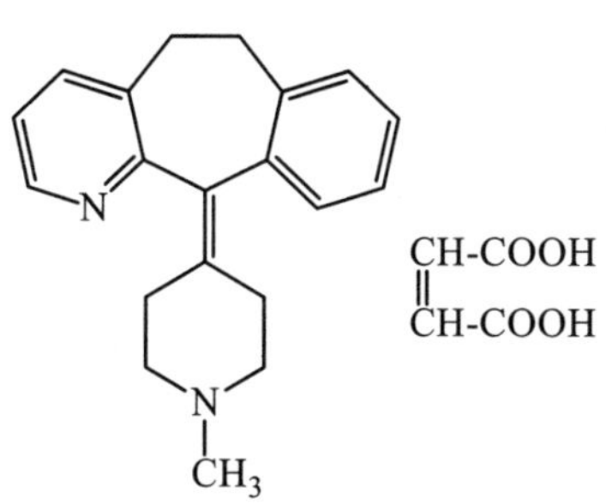

1 1 - (1 - Methyl piperine - 4 - ylidene) - 6, 11 - dihydro - 5H - benzo - [5, 6] - cyclohepata [1, 2-b] - pyridine but - 2 - enedioic acid

It is an antihistamine, related to Cyproheptadine, with anti-serotonin, sedative and anticholinergic effects. It is an azo isomer of Cyproheptadine in which 10 and 11 double bond is reduced which gives a potent, low sedative compound.

Mechanism of action: It is a H_1 antagonists act by competing with histamine for H_1-receptor sites and reduces the intensity of allergic reactions and tissue injury response involving histamine release.

Use: It possess antihistaminic, anticholinergic, antiserotonin and sedative properties. It is used in the treatment of rhinitis, urticaria and other mild allergic conditions.

3.5.2 SECOND GENERATION ANTIHISTAMINES

Second-generation histamine H_1 receptor antagonists have been developed to reduce or eliminate the sedation and anticholinergic adverse effects that occur with older H_1 receptor antagonists.

Mechanism of action: Both first- and second-generation antihistamines are competitive antagonists to histamine at the H_1 receptor site. First generation antihistamines antagonize the acetylcholine at neuronal and neuromuscular muscarinic receptors. But second-generation antihistamine binds only to peripheral H_1 receptor and with no sedation. Because of poor CNS penetration and lower affinity for central histaminic, cholinergic and adrenergic receptors they have no central action like sedation. They are used for the treatment of allergic reactions.

These classes of drugs are divided into two typ ··

(i) Piperazine derivative: eg. Cetirizine

(ii) Pyridine and piperidine derivatives: eg. Loratadine, Fexofenadine, Astemizole.

3.5.2.1 Piperazine Derivative

A. Cetirizine (Tancet, Oncet)

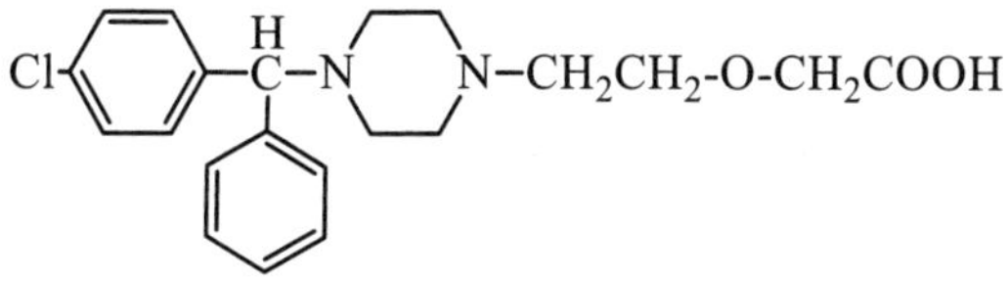

2 - {4 - [(4 - Chloro phenyl) phenyl methyl] - 1- piperazinyl ethoxy} acetic acid

This compound is a Zwitter ions and relatively polar and thus does not penetrate blood brain barrier. The advantage of this compound is once daily dosing, rapid onset of activity and minimal CNS effect. No cardio toxic effect when co-administered with imidazole antifungal and macrolide antibiotics. It is a racemic compound.

Mechanism of action: It is an orally active and selective second generation H1 receptor antagonist.

Use: It is used to relieve symptom such as itching, sneezing, runny nose and hives.

B. Levocetirizine (Levocet, Vozet)

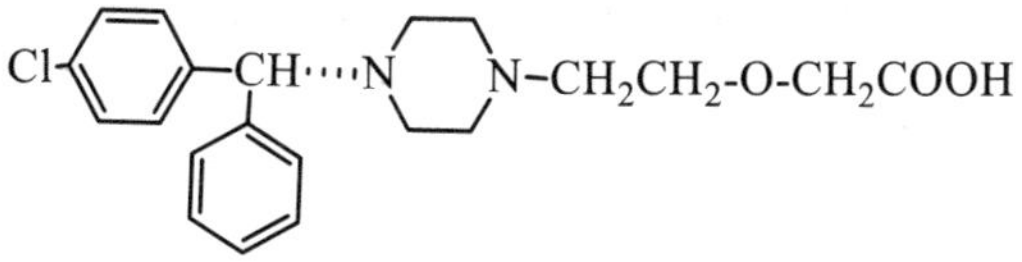

2 - {4R- [(4 - Chloro phenyl) phenyl methyl] - 1- piperazinyl ethoxy} acetic acid

Levocetirizine is R-enantiomer of Cetirizine and display a better pharmacological profile than Cetirizine.

Mechanism of action: Cetirizine are competitive antagonists to histamine peripheral H_1 - receptor

Use: It is used as antihistamine to treat various allergic conditions.

3.5.2.2 Pyridine and Piperidine Derivatives

A. Loratadine (Alastin, Alaspan)

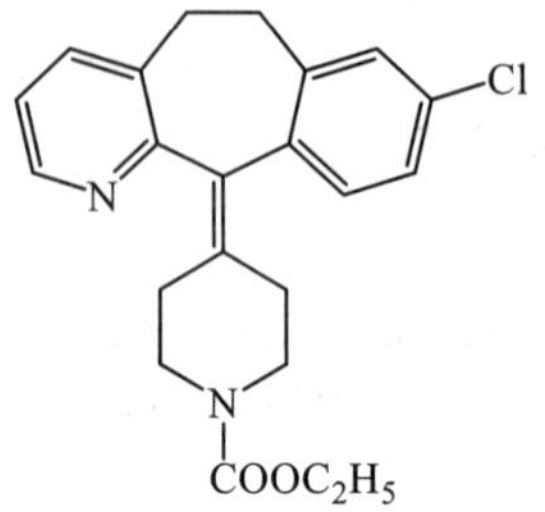

Ethyl 4 - (8 - Chloro - 5, 6 - dihydro -11H - benzo - [5,6] - cyclohepta - [1, 2-b] - pyridin -11 - ylidene) - 1 - piperidin carboxylate

Loratadine is an azo isomer of Cyproheptadine. It is structurally related to Azatadine. The replacement of methyl group of Azatadine (piperidine nitrogen) by corresponding carbamate and introduction of 8-chloro substitutes preserve the antihistaminic action and reduce the CNS effect (Sedative).

Mechanism of action: It binds to H_1 histamine receptors found on the surface of epithelial cells, endothelial cells, eosinophils, neutrophils, airway cells and vascular smooth muscle cells. It prevents severity of histamine mediated symptoms.

Use: It is a potent non-sedating antihistamine used in the treatment of seasonal allergic rhinitis, asthma, conjunctivitis and urticaria.

B. Astemizole (Acemiz, Acipax)

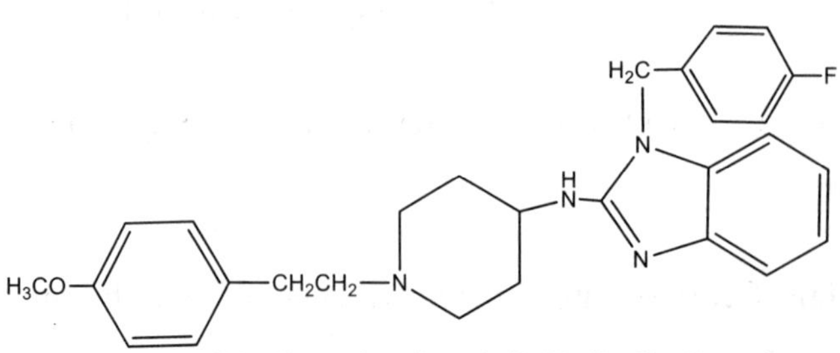

1- [(4 - Fluoro phenyl) methyl] - N - [1 - [2 - (4 -methoxy phenyl) ethyl] piperidin - 4 - yl] benzimidazol - 2 - amine

Mechanism of action: It acts as a reversible competitive inhibitor of histamine H_1-receptor, with less anticholinergic effects compared to related agents.

Use: It is a long-acting, non-sedative antihistamine used in the treatment of seasonal allergic rhinitis, asthma, allergic conjunctivitis and chronic idiopathic urticaria.

3.5.3 H_2 RECEPTOR ANTAGONIST

H_2 antagonists are a type of antihistamine, that block the action of histamine at the histamine H_2 receptors of the parietal cells in the stomach. This decreases the production of stomach acid. H_2 antagonists can be used in the treatment of dyspepsia, peptic ulcers and gastro esophageal reflux disease. They are also called as H_2 blockers. They include, Cimetidine imidazole derivative; Ranitidine substituted furans derivative, Famotidine is a member of the guanidine thiazole group and Roxatidine belongs to the aminoalkyl phenoxy series.

Mechanism of action

The principal stimulants for acid secretion are histamine, gastrin and acetylcholine released from postganglionic enteric neurons. Normally, after a meal, gastrin stimulates the release of histamine, which then binds to histamine H_2 receptors and leads to gastric acid release. H_2 blockers decrease gastric acid secretion by reversibly binding to histamine H_2 receptors located on gastric parietal cells, thereby inhibiting the binding and action of the histamine.H_2 blockers inhibit basal and nocturnal gastric secretion as well as secretion stimulated by food and pentagastrin. H_2 receptor antagonist are used in therapeutic application of acid peptic disorders ranging from heart burn to peptic ulcer disease, Zollinger-Ellison syndrome, gastro oesophageal reflux disease, acute stress ulcers and erosions.

A. Cimetidine (Tagamet)

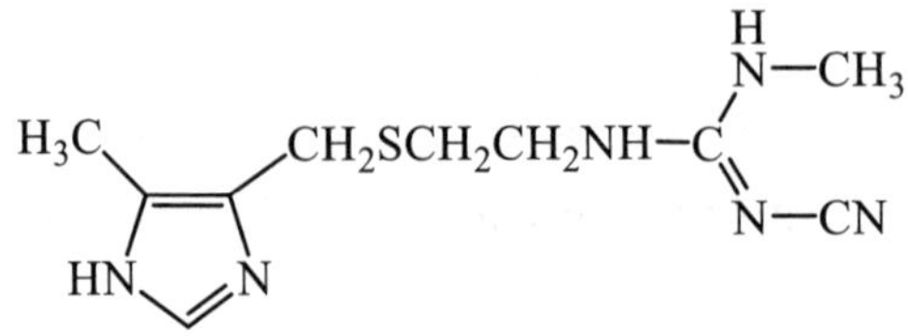

N^1 - Cyano - N^2 - methyl - N^3- {2 - [[(5 - methyl - 1H - imidazol - 4 - yl) methyl]thio]ethyl}guanidine

Synthesis

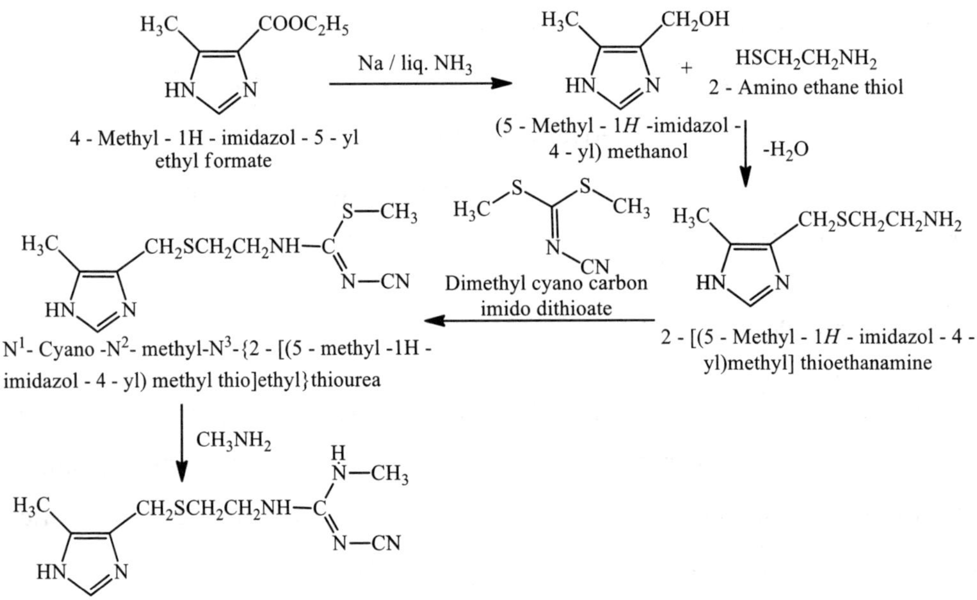

Cimetidine

Mechanism of action: It decrease gastric acid secretion by reversibly binding to histamine H_2 receptors located on gastric parietal cells, thereby inhibiting the binding and action of the histamine. They inhibit basal and nocturnal gastric secretion as well as secretion stimulated by food and pentagastrin.

Use: It is used in gastric and duodenal ulcer.

B. Famotidine (Acilo, Fam)

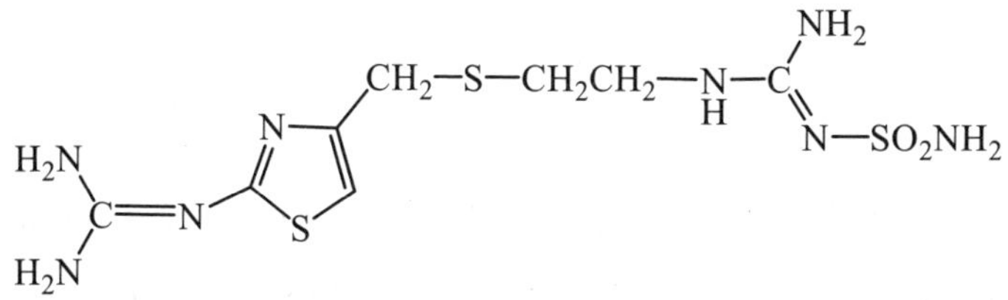

N' - (Amino sulfoxyl) - 3 - [[2 - (diamino methylene)amino] - 4 - thiazolyl] methyl] thio] propionamide

Mechanism of action: It is a competitive inhibitor of histamine H_2 receptors and inhibits basal and nocturnal gastric secretion as well as secretion stimulated by food and pentagastrin.

Use: It is used in the treatment of duodenal and gastric ulcers, Zollinger- Ellison syndrome and heart burn.

C. Ranitidine (Rantac)

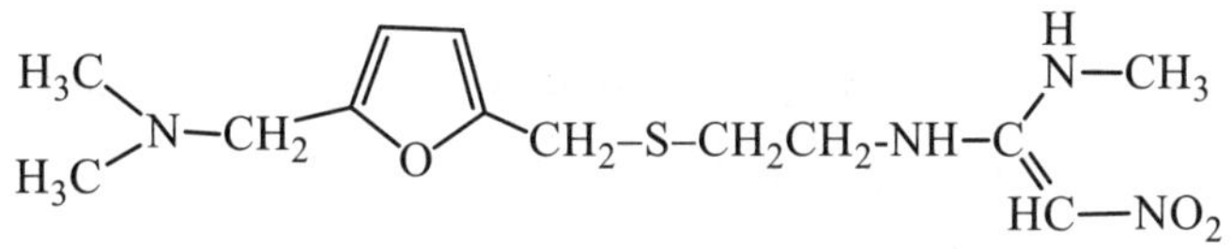

N - [2 -[[[5 - (Dimethyl amino) methyl] - 2 - furanyl] methyl] thio] ethyl] - N' - methyl - 2 - nitro -1, 1 - ethenediamine

Mechanism of action: It decrease gastric acid secretion by reversibly binding to histamine H_2 receptors located on gastric parietal cells, thereby inhibiting the binding and action of the histamine. They inhibit basal and nocturnal gastric secretion as well as secretion stimulated by food and pentagastrin.

Use: It is used in treating duodenal ulcer.

3.5.4 GASTRIC PROTON PUMP INHIBITORS

Gastric proton pump inhibitors (PPIs) are drugs that inhibit the hydrogen/potassium *adenosine triphosphatase* ($H^+K^+ATP_{ase}$) enzyme system of the gastric parietal cells. All PPIs give excellent healing of peptic ulcers and produce good results in reflux esophagitis. PPIs combined with antibiotics eradicate *Helicobacter pylori.*

Mechanism of action

The hydrogen/potassium *adenosine triphosphatase* ($H^+K^+ATP_{ase}$) enzyme normally catalyzes the exchange of H^+ for K^+ at the cell membrane. This is the final stage of acid secretory process, called the pump. Therefore, these drugs antagonize all stimulation (histamine, gastrin, Ach mediated) of the gastric secretion. Proton pump inhibitors are weak bases that act as prodrug and need an acidic environment in order to inhibit the $H^+K^+ATP_{ase}$. All these compounds share a common structure consisting of substituted pyridyl methyl sulfinyl benzimidazoles that varies in terms of the substitutions on either the pyridine or the benzimidazole rings. These drugs become protonated and converted into the active sulfonamide species, which forms disulfide bonds with cysteine residues in the α-subunit of the $H^+K^+ATP_{ase}$. This result in an inhibitory mechanism that is independent of histamine, acetylcholine or gastrin stimulus for acid secretion. Decreasing the acid in the stomach can aid the healing of duodenal ulcers and reduce the pain from indigestion and heartburn.

A. Omeprazole (Prilosec)

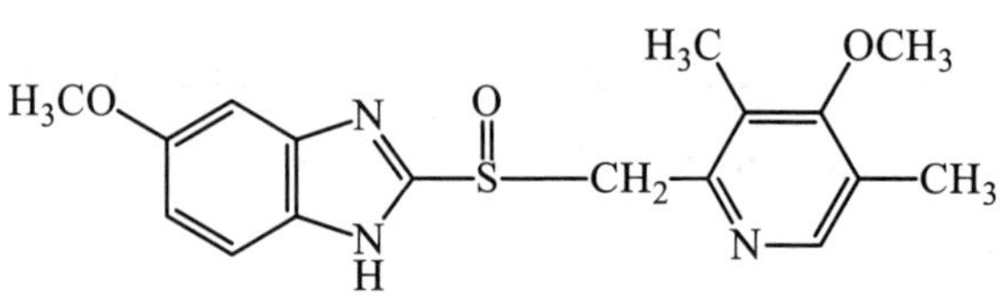

5 - Methoxy - 2 - (((4 - methoxy - 3, 5 - dimethyl - 2 - pyridinyl) methyl) sulfinyl) - 1H - benzimidazole

Use: It is used in the treatment of duodenal ulcer, gastric ulcer and pathological hypersecretory conditions.

B. Lansoprazole (Prevacid)

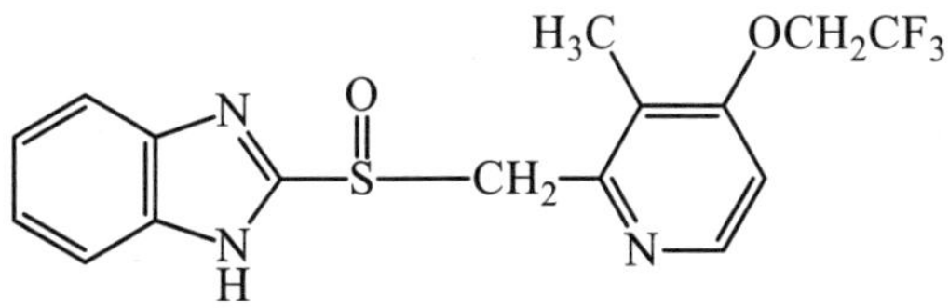

2 - [[(3 - Methyl - 4 - (2, 2, 2 - trifluoro ethoxy) - 2 - pyridyl) methyl) sulfinyl] benzimidazole

Use: It is used in the treatment and prevention of NSAID-induced gastric ulcers as well as Zollinger-Ellison syndrome.

C. Pantoprazole (Protonix)

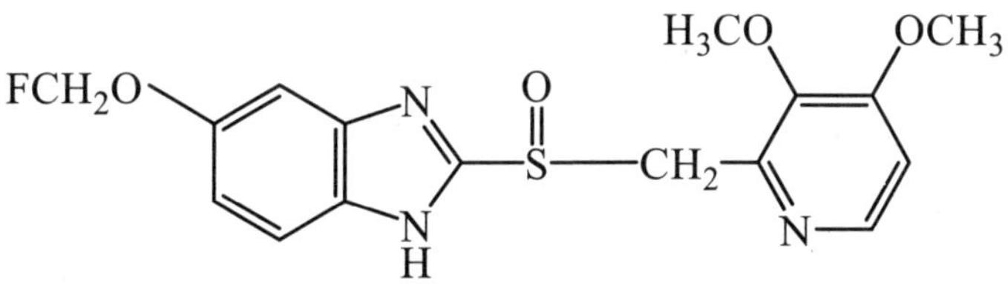

5 - (Difluoro methoxy) - 2 - [[3, 4 - dimethoxy - 2 - pyridinyl) methyl) sulfinyl] - 1H - benzimidazole

Use: It is used in the treatment of pathological hypersecretory conditions associated with Zollinger-Ellison syndrome.

D. Rabeprazole (Aciphex)

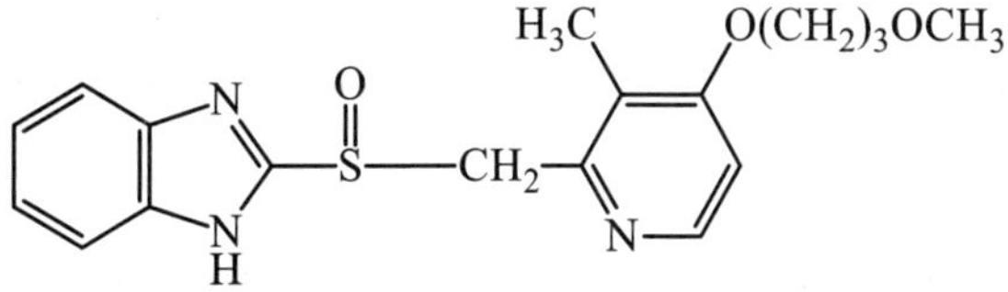

2 - [[[4 - (3 - Methoxy propoxy) - 3 - methyl - 2 - pyridinyl] methyl] sulfinyl] - 1H - benzimidazole

Use: It is used in gastric hypersecretory disorder.

Chapter 2

ANTINEOPLASTIC AGENTS

1. INTRODUCTION

Antineoplastic agents are the drugs used in the treatment of cancer, malignancy, tumour, carcinoma, sarcoma, leukaemia etc., Cancer is a term used for diseases in which abnormal cells divide without control and are able to invade other tissues. The term neoplasm refers to an abnormal mass of tissue arising from an abnormal proliferation of cells. The body is made up of trillions of cells that grow, divide and die in an orderly fashion. This process is regulated by DNA within the cell. When a person is growing up, the cells of the body rapidly divide, but once adulthood is reached, cells generally divide to replace worn-out, dying cells or to repair injured cells. When these cells proliferate in an abnormal manner, that is not coordinated with the surrounding tissue as this excessive growth persists, a lump or tumour is usually formed. Based on the functions/locations of the cells from which they originate cancer is categorized as:

- **Carcinoma:** skin or in tissues that line or cover internal organs. eg. Epithelial cells. 80-90% reported cancer cases are carcinomas.
- **Sarcoma:** bone, cartilage, fat, muscle, blood vessels or other connective or supportive tissue.
- **Leukaemia:** white blood cells and their precursor cells such as bone marrow cells, causes large numbers of abnormal blood cells to be produced and enter the blood.
- **Lymphoma:** cells of the immune system that affect lymphatic system.
- **Myeloma:** B-cells that produces antibodies-spreads through lymphatic system.
- **Central nervous system cancers:** cancers that begin in the tissues of the brain and spinal cord.

2. CLASSIFICATION

Antineoplastic agents are classified according to their mechanism of action into:

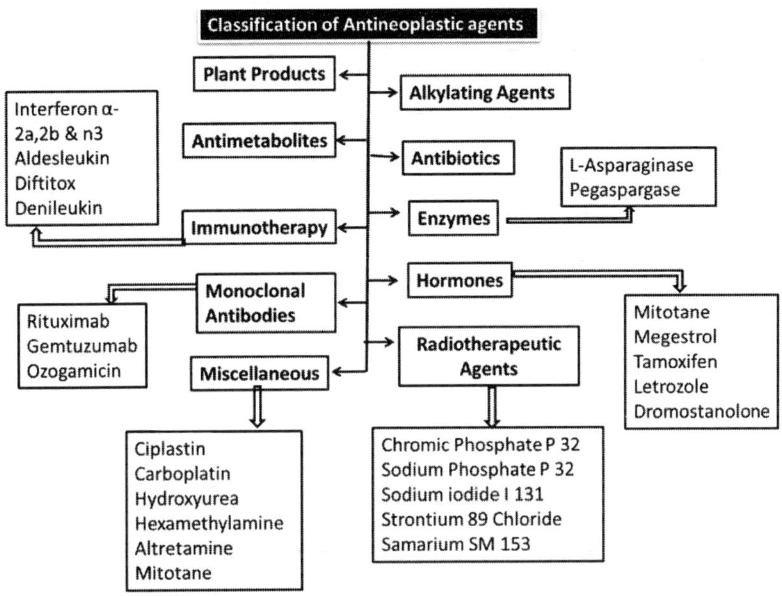

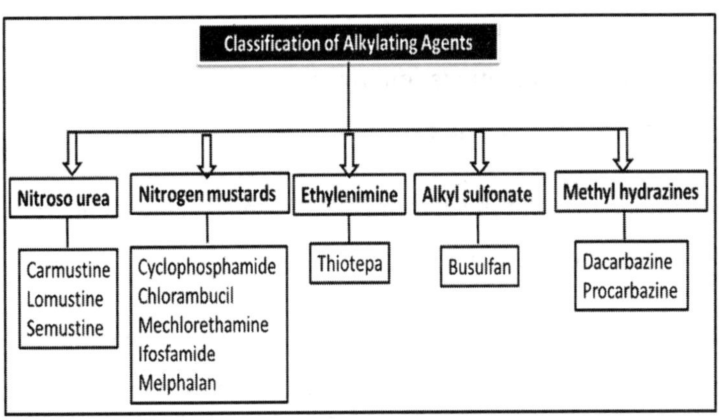

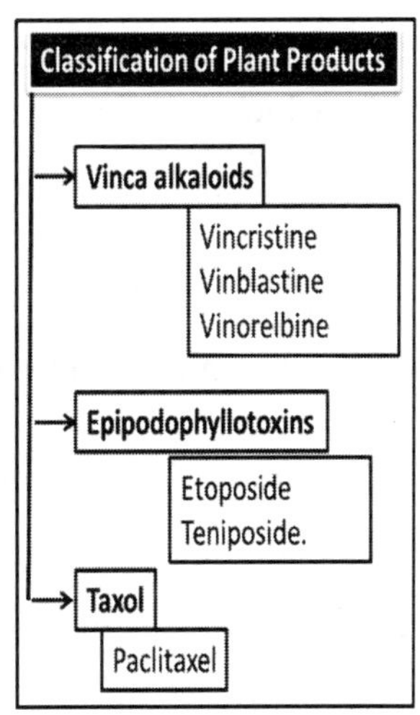

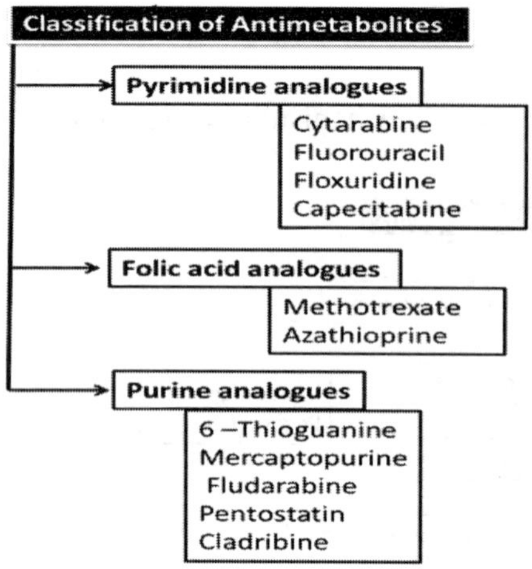

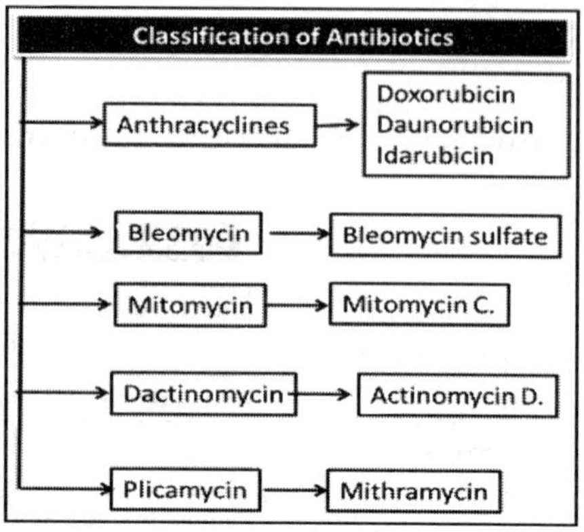

2.1 Alkylating Agents

Alkylating agents are so named because of their ability to add alkyl groups to many electronegative groups under conditions present in cells. They stop tumor growth by cross-linking guanine bases in DNA double-helix strands - directly attacking DNA. This makes the strands unable to uncoil and separate. As this is necessary in DNA replication, the cells can no longer divide. In addition, these drugs add methyl or other alkyl groups onto molecule which in turn inhibits their correct utilization by base pairing and causes a miscoding of DNA. Alkylating agents are cell cycle nonspecific.

Alkylating agents work by three different mechanisms all of which achieve the same end result - disruption of DNA function and cell death

i) Miscoding: The guanine base usually exists as the keto tautomer and base pairs with cytosine. Once alkylated, guanine prefers the enol tautomer and is more likely to base pair with thymine. Such miscoding leads to an alteration in the amino acid sequence of protein which in turn leads to disruption of protein structure and function.

ii) Alkylating agent may also link with 2-guanine group on the same chain such that the drug is attached like a limpet to the side of the DNA helix. Such an attachment would mask that portion of DNA and block access to the necessary enzymes required for DNA function.

iii) It may also lead to the cleavage of imidazole ring in guanine which destroys guanine.

Under physiological condition, alkylating agents are positively charged (electrophile) and they react with negative or high electron density region. They act by alkylating N - 7 position of guanine in DNA, which results in the formation of apurinic site. The alkylating agent appears to be most effective in G_1 or S phase

$$\underset{\text{Nucleophile or Bioploymer}}{\text{nu - H}} + \underset{\text{Alkylating agent}}{\text{alkyl - Y}} \longrightarrow \text{alkyl - nu} + \overset{\oplus}{H} + \overset{\ominus}{Y}$$

Leaving group is chloride in Mechlorethamine, Cyclophosphamide and Melphalan and methylsulfonate in Busulfan. There are five groups of alkylating agents includes, nitrogen mustard, nitroso urea, methyl hydrazines, ethylenimines and alkyl sulfonates.

2.1.1 Nitrogen Mustards

A. Mechlorethamine (Mustargen, Mustine)

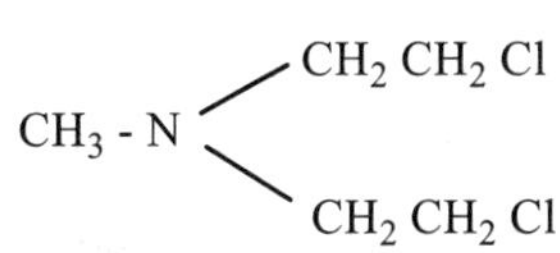

2, 2' - Dichloro - N - methyl diethylamine

Synthesis

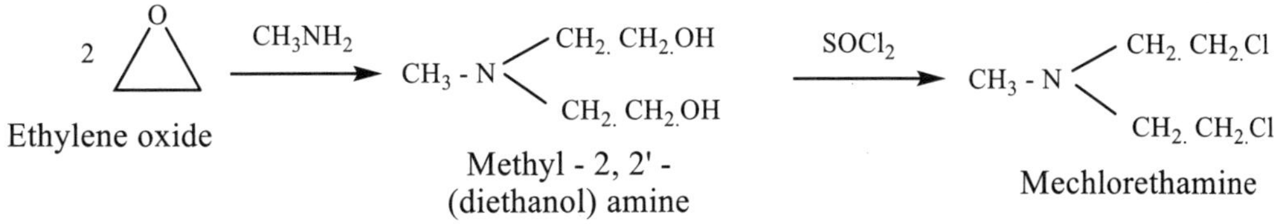

Mechanism of action: At physiological pH, aliphatic nitrogen mustard converts into stable aziridinium ion, which once produced reacts with nucleophilic center in the biomolecule. The nitrogen mustard is quite reactive agent and administered intravenously. The nitrogen atom can displace a chloride ion intramolecularly to form a highly electrophilic aziridinium ion. (Fig.2.1)

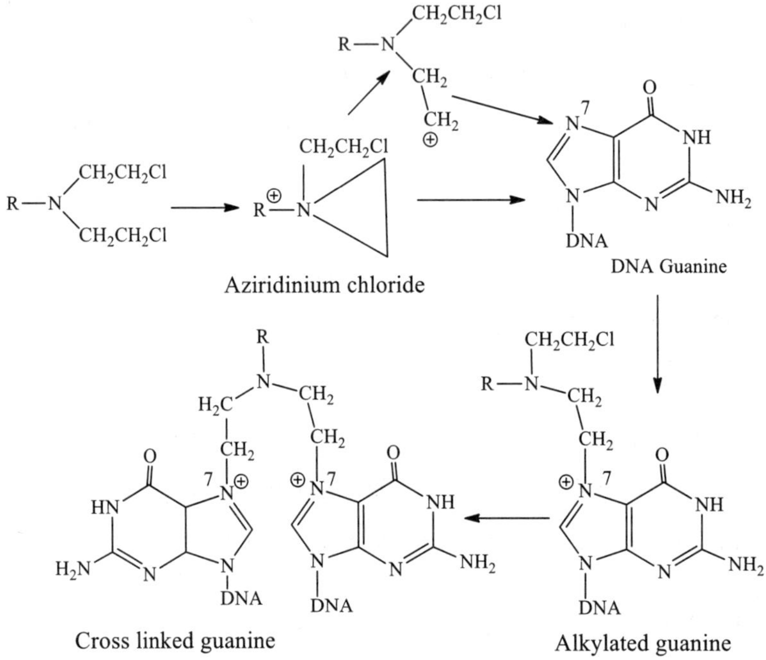

Fig. 2.1 General Mechanism of Alkylating Agents

Aryl substituted nitrogen mustard such as Chlorambucil and amide-like phosphoramide linkages Cyclophosphamide are relatively stable to aziridinium ion formation because the aromatic ring decreases the nucleophilicity of the nitrogen atom. This stability allows it to be taken orally, whereas Mechlorethamine is given intravenously.

Use: It is used in Hodgkin's disease. It is used in combination with Vincristine, Procarbazine and Prednisone.

B. Cyclophosphamide (Cyphos, Oncomide)

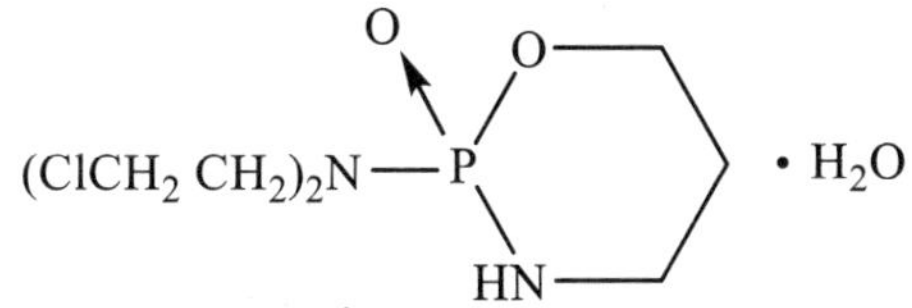

2 - [Bis (2 - chloro ethyl) amino] tetrahydro - 2H - 1, 3, 2 - oxazo - phosphorin - 2 - oxide monohydrate

Cyclophosphamide has advantage over another alkylating agent, in that it is active orally and parenterally. It requires metabolic activation (prodrug).

Mechanism of action

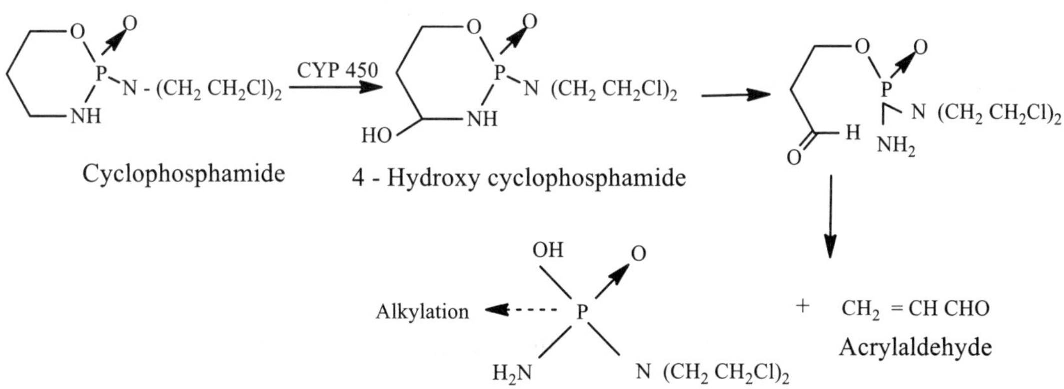

Fig. 2.2 Metabolic Activation of Cyclophosphamide

Bio-activation by CYP450 enzyme gives hydroxylation to an unstable carbinolamine intermediate. This undergoes non-enzymatic fragmentation to acrylaldehyde and phosphoramide mustard which acts as alkylating agent. (Fig. 2.2)

Use: It is used against multiple myeloma, chronic lymphocytic leukaemia and acute leukaemia of children.

C. Melphalan (Alkacel, Alkeran)

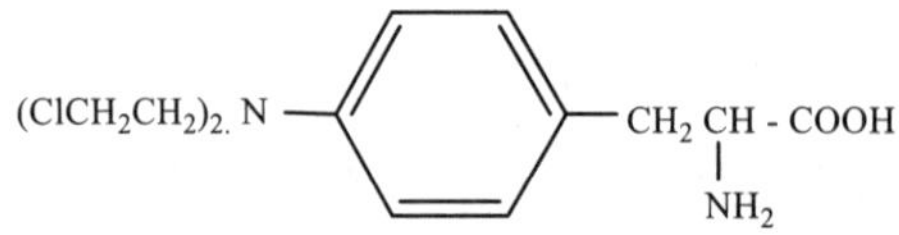

4 - [Bis (2 - chloro ethyl) amino] - L - phenyl alanine

The *levo* isomer of Melphalan is used as alkylating agent and *dextro* isomer of Melphalan is toxic to bone marrow and carcinogenic.

Mechanism of action: It alkylates DNA at the N-7 position of guanine and induces DNA inter-strand cross-linkages, resulting in inhibition of DNA and RNA synthesis.

Use: It is active against multiple myeloma, breast, testicular and ovarian carcinoma.

D. Chlorambucil (Leukeran)

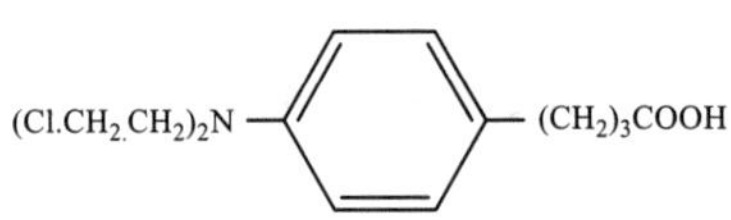

4 - {p - [Bis(2 - chloro ethyl) amino] phenyl} butyric acid

It acts slowly, so less toxic than any other nitrogen mustard derivatives in use.

Mechanism of action: Alkylation takes place through the formation of a highly reactive ethylenimonium radical and forms a cross-linkage between two strands of DNA, interfering with DNA, RNA and protein synthesis.

Use: It is used in the treatment of chronic lymphocytic leukaemia (CLL), macroglobulinemia, lymphosarcoma and Hodgkin's disease.

2.1.2 Alkylsolfonate

A. Busulfan (Bucelan, Mylefan)

$CH_3SO_2O\ (CH_2)_4OSO_2CH_3$

1, 4 - Bis (methane sulfonyloxy) butane

It is an alkyl sulphonic acid ester. It is a methane sulfonate diester of 1, 4-butanediol.

Mechanism of action: It is a bifunctional alkylating agent. It destroys cancerous cells by interfering with the DNA in cancer cells, via intrastrand crosslinks thereby preventing them from further dividing and ultimately leading to cell death through apoptosis. Methanesulfonate eliminated as a leaving group.

Use: Busulfan is used in the treatment of chronic granulocytic leukaemia.

2.1.3 Ethylenimine

A. Thiotepa (Thioplex)

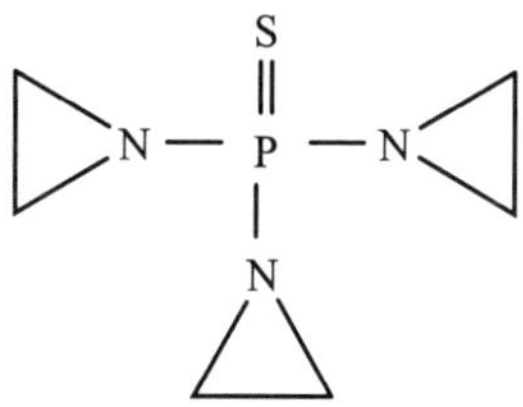

Tri - (1- aziridinyl) phosphine sulfide

Thiotepa is an aziridine containing drug.

Mechanism of Action: At acidic pH, the aziridine group is protonated to provide a reactive aziridinium ion that is known to alkylate DNA.

Use: It is used in the treatment of variety of tumours, breast, ovarian and bronchogenic carcinoma and malignant lymphomas.

2.2 Antimetabolites

Antimetabolites are compounds that prevent the biosynthesis or use of normal cellular metabolite. Chemical substances, which take part in cellular metabolites, are called antimetabolites. Antimetabolites exert their action by acting as a false precursor for enzyme or by acting as a competitive antagonist for an enzyme. These drugs are usually structural analogues of normal body metabolite, derived by incorporating one or two bio-isosteric group or other structural changes of the metabolite. They compete with the natural substrate for the active site on an essential enzyme or receptor. Some are incorporated directly into DNA or RNA. Most are phase-specific, acting during the S-phase of the cell cycle. Their efficacy is usually greater over a prolonged period, so they are usually given continuously. There are three main classes namely Pyrimidine analogues, Purine analogues and Folic acid analogues.

2.2.1 Pyrimidine Analogues

The structural modification of these metabolites may be on the pyrimidine ring. These drugs resemble pyrimidine molecules and work by either, inhibiting the synthesis of nucleic acids or incorporated into DNA, which interferes with DNA synthesis and resulting in cell death.

A. Fluorouracil (Flocil)

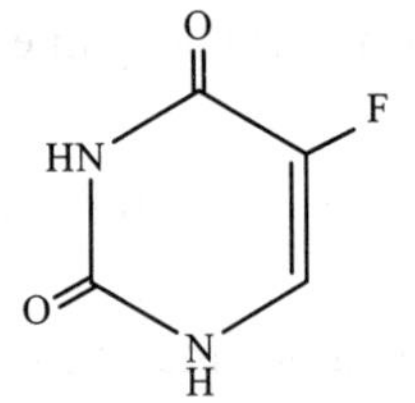

5 - Fluoro - 2, 4 - (1H, 3H) pyrimidinedione

Mechanism of action: Fluorouracil is an analog of the pyrimidine uracil and thus acts as a pyrimidine antagonist. It interferes with DNA synthesis by blocking the *thymidylate synthetase* enzyme involved in the synthesis of thymidine.

There are three possible mechanisms of action

- Fluorouracil metabolite fluorodeoxyuridine monophosphate competes with uracil to bind with *thymidylate synthetase* and folate cofactor. This result in, decreased thymidine production and therefore decreased DNA synthesis and repair and ultimately decreased cell proliferation.

- Fluorouracil metabolite fluorodeoxyuridine triphosphate is incorporated into DNA thus interfering with DNA replication.
- Fluorouracil metabolite fluorouridine-5-triphosphate is incorporated into RNA in place of uridine triphosphate (dUTP), producing a false RNA and interfering with RNA processing and protein synthesis. It results in mutation and in cell death.

Use: Fluorouracil is effective in the palliative management of carcinoma of the breast, colon, pancreas, rectum and stomach in patient who cannot be cured by surgery. It is also used in the treatment of skin and basal cell carcinomas.

B. Floxuridine (FUDR)

Floxuridine is a prodrug of 5-Fluorouracil. It is freely soluble in water than 5-Fluorouracil. Metabolically the deoxy sugar moiety of Floxuridine is cleaved to give 5-Fluorouracil.

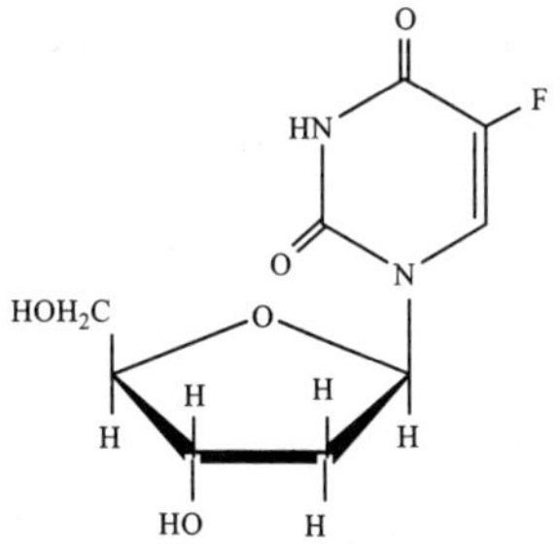

1 - (2 - Deoxy - β - D - ribofuranosyl) - 5 - fluorouracil

Mechanism of action: Metabolically the deoxy sugar moiety of Floxuridine is cleaved to give 5-Fluorouracil which acts by interfering with DNA synthesis.

Use: It is used for gastrointestinal adenocarcinoma.

C. Cytarabine (Aracid, Cytabin)

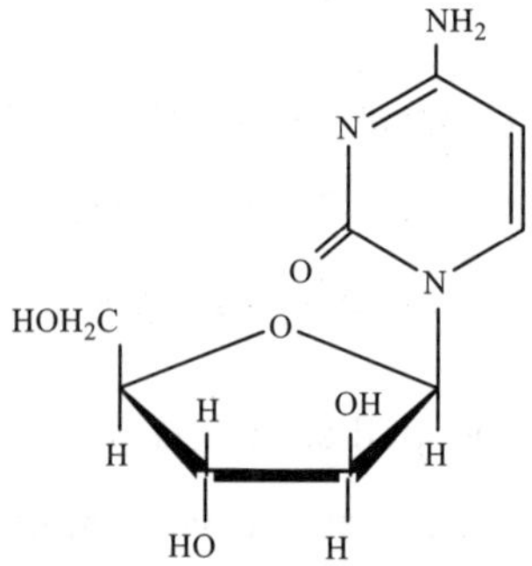

1 - β - D -Arabino furanosyl cytosine

Cytarabine is an example of pyrimidine antimetabolite in which the sugar has been modified and also known as cytosine arabinoside (Ara-C). Cytarabine combines a cytosine base with an arabinose sugar. In this case, the sugar moiety arabinose with 2' - OH group has β-configuration rather than the normal α-configuration.

Mechanism of action: Cytarabine is metabolized intracellularly into its active triphosphate form (cytosine arabinoside triphosphate). This metabolite then damages DNA by acting as a competitive inhibitor of *DNA polymerase* an enzyme that synthesizes DNA molecules from deoxyribonucleotides. Incorporation of cytosine arabinoside triphosphate into DNA chain, leads to miscoding. It is specific for the S-phase of the cell cycle.

Use: It is used for acute leukaemia, chronic myelocytic leukaemia, meningeal leukaemia, acute lympholytic leukaemia and chronic lympholytic leukaemia. Cytarabine also possesses antiviral activity and used for the treatment of generalized herpes virus infection

2.2.2 Purine Analogues

These are analogues of natural purine bases and nucleotides. 6-Mercaptopurine (6MP) and Thioguanine are derivatives of adenine and guanine respectively. A sulphur group replaces the keto group on C_6 in these compounds. In many cases, the drugs require initial activation. They are then able to inhibit nucleotide biosynthesis by direct incorporation into DNA.

A. Mercaptopurine (Purineton)

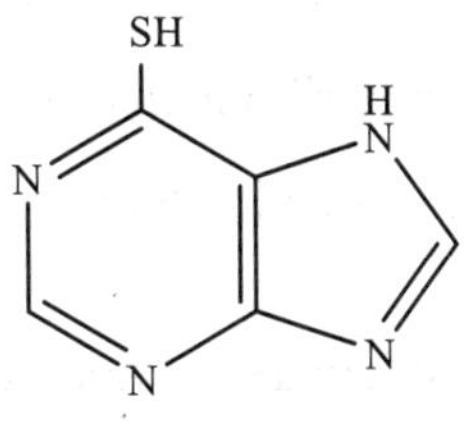

Purine - 6 - thiol

Synthesis

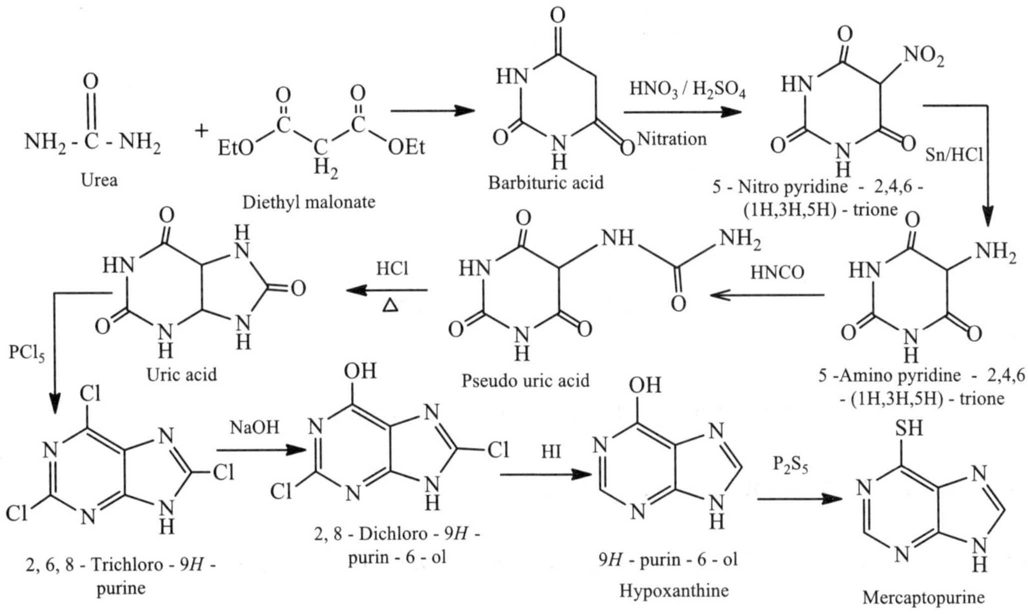

Mechanism of action: Mercaptopurine interferes with nucleic acid synthesis by inhibiting purine metabolism. It is a pro-drug that is converted intracellularly metabolized according to the following ways

- Mercaptopurine is first converted to thioinosine monophosphate (TIMP) by the enzyme *hypoxanthine-guanine phosphoribosyl transferase*. TIMP inhibits purine synthesis.
- The TIMP sequentially phosphorylated into diphosphate and triphosphate which is incorporated into RNA and DNA. This results in non-functional RNA and DNA.

- Upon methylation, TIMP forms 6-methylthioinosinate (MTIMP) which inhibits *glutamine-5-phosphoribosyl pyrophosphate amido transferase,* first enzyme unique to the *de novo* pathway for purine ribonucleotide synthesis. TIMP methylation is an effective inhibitor of *de novo* purine biosynthesis.

Use: It is used to treat myelomonocytic leukaemia and non-Hodgkin's lymphoma.

B. Azathioprine (Imuran)

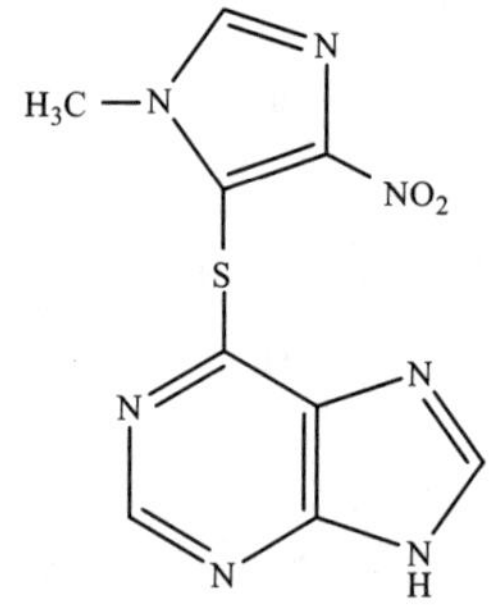

6 - [(1 - Methyl - 4 - nitro -1H - imidazol - 5 - yl) thio] -1H - purine.

Azathioprine acts as a prodrug for Mercaptopurine.

Mechanism of action: Same as Mercaptopurine

Use: It is converted into 6-Mercaptopurine and possess similar use as 6-MP.

C. Thioguanine (Tabloid)

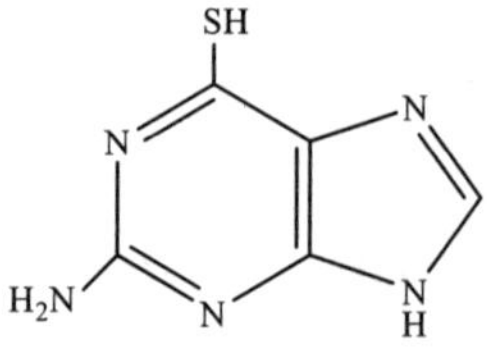

2 - Amino purine - 6 - thiol

Mechanism of action: It is converted *by hypoxanthine-guanine phosphoribosyl transferase* into a nucleotide form, which inhibits a number of reactions in DNA and RNA synthesis.

Use: It is used in the treatment of acute leukaemia, in combination with Cytarabine.

2.2.3 Folic acid Analogues

Folic acid analogues act by inhibiting the metabolism of folic acid. Folic acid is needed for the *de novo* synthesis of nucleoside required for DNA synthesis. Folic acid antagonists kill cells by inhibiting DNA synthesis in the S-phase of the cell cycle.

A. Methotrexate (Oncotrex, Plastomet)

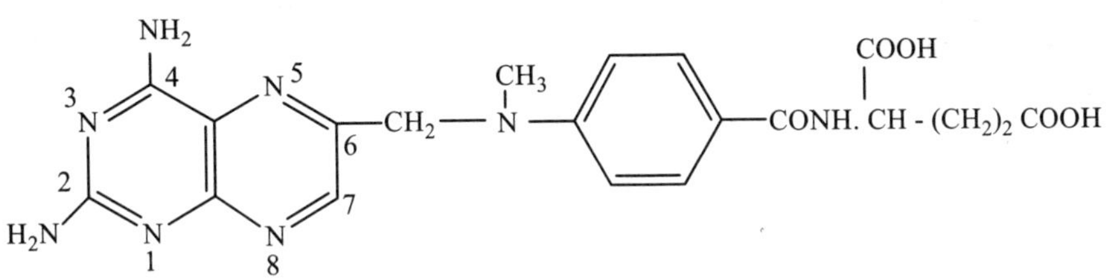

N - [4 - [[(2, 4 - diamino - 6 - pteridinyl) methyl] methylamino] benzoyl] - L - glutamic acid

Synthesis

Step I: Synthesis of 6-(Bromomethyl) pteridine - 2, 4 - diamine

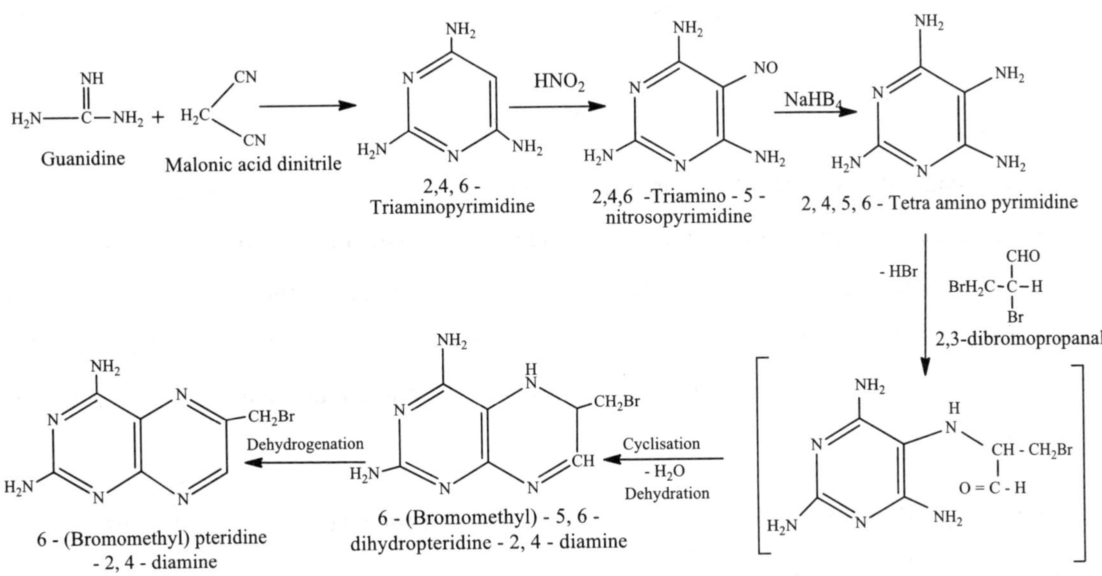

Step II: Synthesis of N-(4-Methylaminobenzoyl) glutamic acid

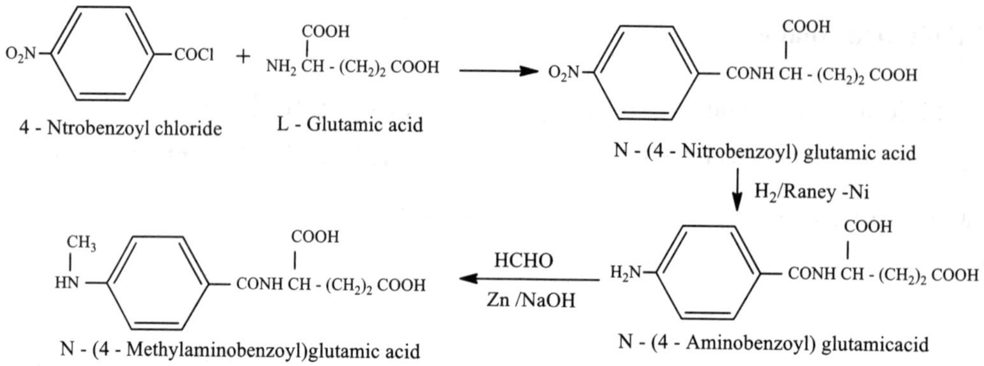

Step III: Synthesis of Methotrexate

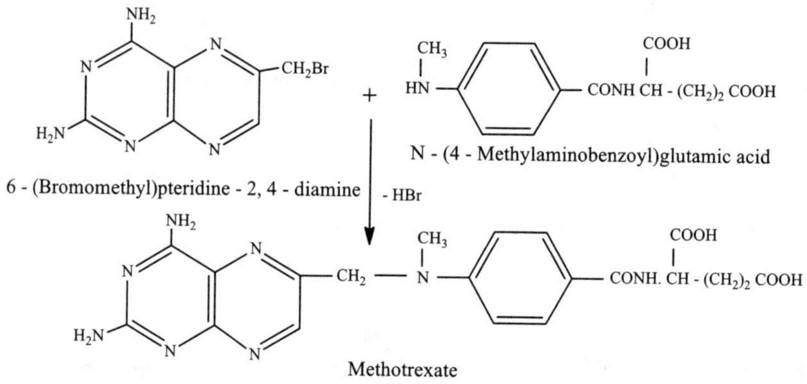

Mechanism of action: It competitively inhibits *dihydrofolate reductase*, which is responsible for the formation of tetrahydrofolate from dihydrofolic acid. This is essential for the generation of a variety of coenzymes that are involved in the synthesis of purines, thymidylate, methionine and glycine. Methotrexate, therefore, inhibits the synthesis of DNA and RNA thymidylates and proteins. Inhibition of nucleotide synthesis prevents cell division.

Use: It is used against leukaemia, lymphoma, lung and osteosarcoma. It is also used in the treatment of rheumatoid arthritis.

2.3 Antibiotics

2.3.1 Anthracycline

Anthracyclines are large and complex family of antibiotics. Anthracyclines from both natural and semisynthetic sources are most widely used chemotherapeutic agents and are effective against a broad spectrum of solid tumors and leukemias. They are extracted from *Streptomyces* bacterium.

They occur as glycoside of the anthracyclinone attached by a glycosidic linkage to the amino sugar daunosamine. Anthracyclinone refers to an aglycone containing the anthraquinone chromophore with a linear hydrocarbon skeleton related to that of tetracycline sugar. Because of the conjugated anthraquinone nucleus, the anthracylines are red in color and impart a red color to the urine of the patient. The glycosidic linkage usually involves the 7 - hydroxy group of the anthracyclinone and β- anomer of sugar with L – configurations.

Anthracycline derivatives that differ by the substitution patterns on the anthraquinone segment or by the sugar unit vary in their spectrum of antitumor activity and dose-limiting cardiotoxicity.

Mechanism of action: Anthracycline has three mechanisms of action:

- Inhibit DNA and RNA synthesis by intercalating between base pairs of the DNA/RNA strand, thus preventing the replication of rapidly growing cancer cells.
- Inhibit *topoisomerase - II* enzyme, preventing the relaxing of supercoiled DNA and thus blocking DNA transcription and replication.
- Creates free oxygen radicals such as hydroxyl radical and super oxide radical anion. These free radicals may produce destructive effect upon the cell which may include damage of DNA. The generation of free radicals leads to cardio toxicity, a major side effect of anthracycline.

Clinically the most important anthracyclines are Doxorubicin, Daunorubicin, Idarubicin and Epirubicin. Due to lack of oral activity all the anthracyclines are administered intravenously.

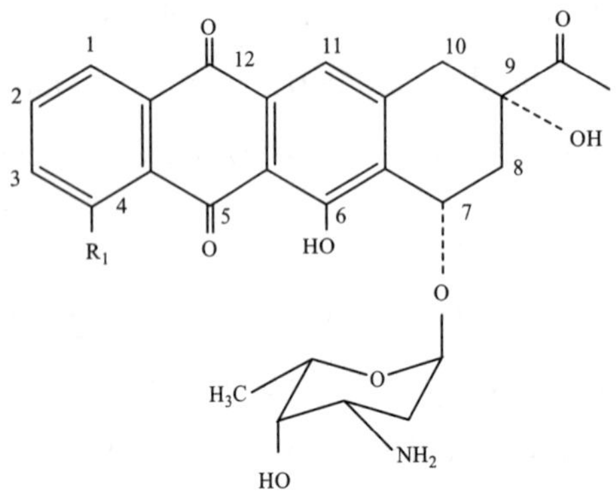

Name	R_1	R_2
Daunorubicin	$-OCH_3$	-H
Doxorubicin	$-OCH_3$	-OH

A. Daunorubicin (Daunomycin, Daunoside)

Daunorubicin is obtained from fermentation of *Streptomyces peucetius*. It is a glycoside formed between daunomycin and L-daunosamine.

Use: It is used in the treatment of acute lymphocytic and granulocytic leukemias.

B. Doxorubicin (Oncodex, Epricin)

Doxorubicin is 14-Hydroxydaunorubicin obtained from the cultures of *Streptomyces peucetius*. It is the one of the most effective antitumor agent. Doxorubicin has been used in acute lymphoblastic and myeloblastic leukaemia, Wilms' tumor, neuroblastoma, soft tissue and bone sarcomas, breast, ovarian, thyroid, gastric carcinoma, Hodgkin's disease, malignant lymphoma and bronchogenic carcinoma.

Use: It is used for treatment solid tumors such as breast, thyroid, ovary, bladder and lung cancer, sarcomas and neuroblastoma.

2.3.2 Bleomycin (Bleocip, Oncobleo)

Bleomycin is a mixture of a glycopeptide antitumour antibiotic isolated from the strain of *Streptomyces verticillus*. The main component is Bleomycin A_2 and Bleomycin B_2.

Natural Bleomycin occurs as a copper chelates with ligands provided by the pyrimidine, imidazole, amide and amine functional groups. Although the copper is removed from the pharmaceutical form, metal chelate is the key to antitumor activity.

Mechanism of action: Inside the cell, the Bleomycin forms a chelate with Fe (II) and molecular oxygen. The resulting complex may give rise to hydroxy radical and superoxide radical. These radicals degrade the DNA by reacting with it.

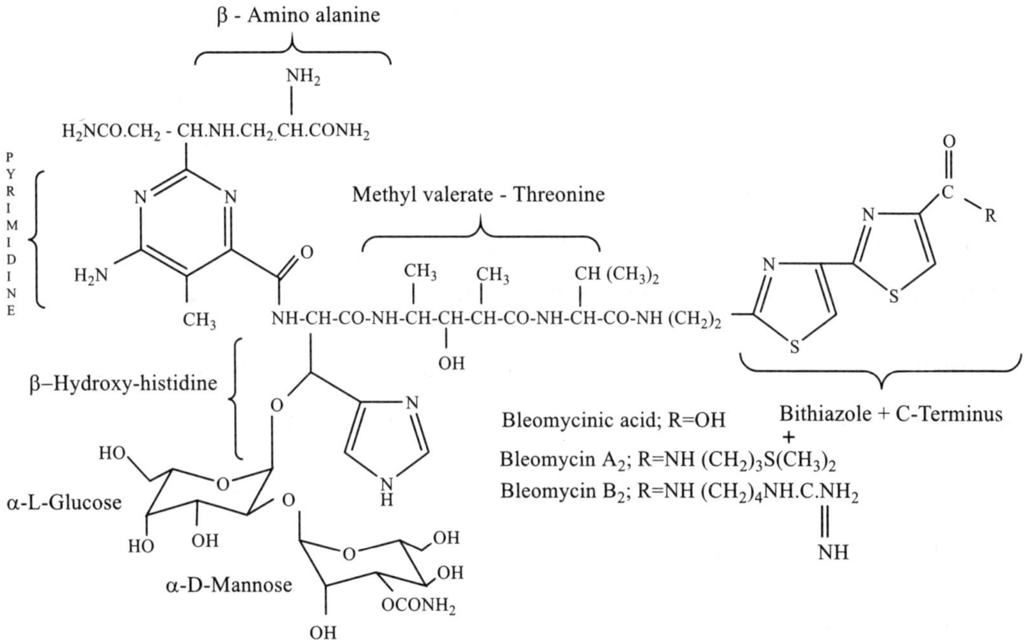

Use: It is used for carcinoma of cervix, head and neck, larynx, penis, skin, testes, Hodgkin's and non-Hodgkin's lymphoma.

2.3.3 Dactinomycin (or) Actinomycin D (Cosmegen, Dacilon)

An example of antineoplastic actinomycin is Dactinomycin

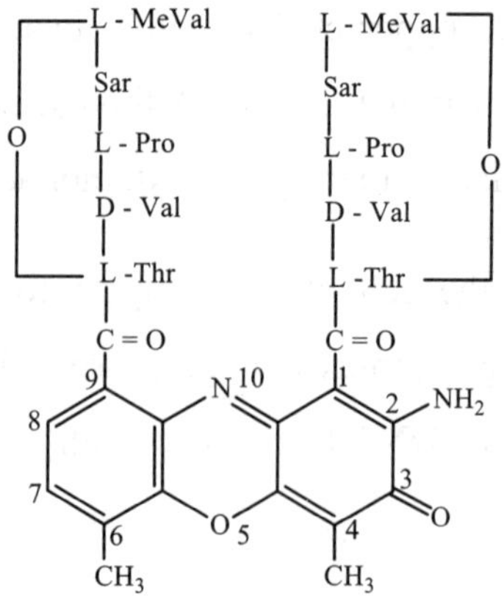

Dactinomycin

It is obtained from the fermentation of selected strains of *Streptomyces parvulus*. It consists of tricyclic phenoxazone ring in the quinone oxidation state and two identical polypeptide lactone appendages. The polypeptides are made up of L-proline and L-threonine plus the non-essential amino acids D-valine, sarcosine and N-methyl valine.

Mechanism of action: This ring system is aromatic and planar and intercalate into DNA at base pair step. This interferes with its replication and transcription.

Use: It is used against carcinoma in testes, Ewing's sarcoma, Trophoblastic tumor, Wilm's tumor and sarcoma botryoides.

2.4 Plant Products

2.4.1 Vinca Alkaloids

The vinca alkaloids are anti-mitotic and anti-microtubule alkaloid agents. The compounds are isolated from the periwinkle *Catharanthus rosea* (*Vinca rosea*). They are composed of two multi ringed units vidoline and catharanthine. Four closely related compounds are, Vincristine, Vinblastine, Vinrosidine and Vinleurosine and semi-synthetic derivative Vinorelbine. Among them, **Vincristine** and **Vinblastine** are important clinical agents.

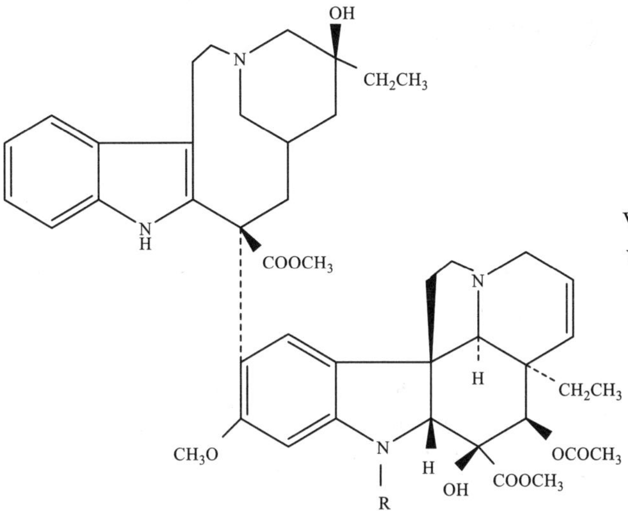

Vincristine: R = CHO

Vinblastine: R = CH_3

Mechanism of action: Vinca alkaloids act as antimicrotubular agents that block mitosis by arresting cells in the metaphase. These drugs act by preventing the polymerization of tubulin to form microtubules, as well as inducing depolymerization of formed tubules. Vinca alkaloids are cell cycle phase-specific for M phase and S phase.

Use: They are effective in acute leukaemia, Hodgkin's, non-Hodgkin's lymphoma, Wilm's tumor and mycosis fungoides.

2.4.2 Epipodophyllotoxins

A. Etoposide (Beposid, Lestet)

Etoposide is a semi-synthetic derivative of podophyllotoxin commonly known as VP-16. The podophyllotoxin are obtained as extracts of May apple plant. The significant difference between the structure of originally isolated natural product and semi synthetic analogues involve the stereo chemical relationship between the substituents at 1, 4 position. The podophyllotoxin have *cis* stereo chemistry but the synthetic analogue is *trans* configuration.

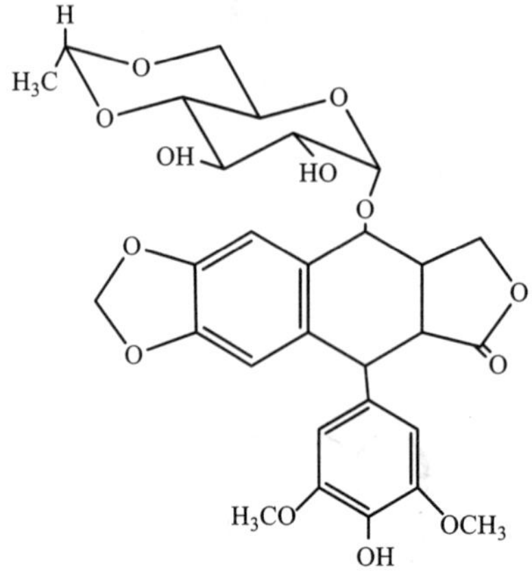

9 - [4, 6 - o - Ethylidene - β – D - gluco pyranosyl) oxy] - 5, 8, 8a, 9 - tetrahydro - 5 - (4' -hydroxy - 3, 5 - dimethoxy phenyl) furo - [3', 4' : 6, 7] - naphtho - [2, 3-d] - 1, 3 - dioxol - 6, 5H - one

Mechanism of action: It inhibits DNA *topoisomerase-II,* thereby kills the cell by stabilizing enzyme-cleaved DNA complex.

Use: It is effective in lung cancer and testicular cancer.

2.5 Hormones

A. Mitotane (Lysodren)

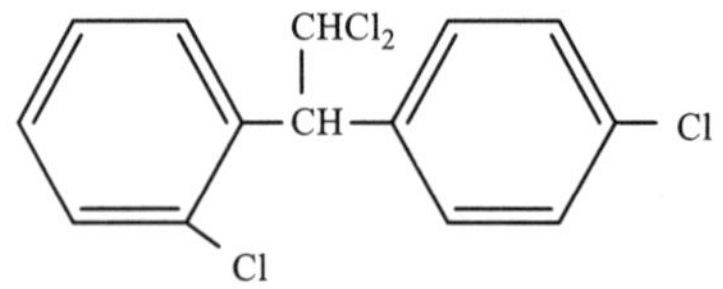

1, 1 - Dichloro - 2 - (o - chloro phenyl) - 2 - (p - chloro phenyl) ethane

Mitotane is an oral adrenal cytotoxic agent. It is structurally related to the insecticide Chlorophenothane (DDT). It is an immunosuppressive agent.

Mechanism of action: It directly suppresses the adrenal cortex, both with and without cellular destruction. Production of corticosteroid is inhibited, and peripheral steroid metabolism is modified, leading to increased excretion of 17-hydroxycorticosteroids and 17-ketosteroids.

Use: It is indicated only for treating adrenal cortex carcinoma.

2.6 Miscellaneous

A. Cisplatin (Cytopaltin, Plationco)

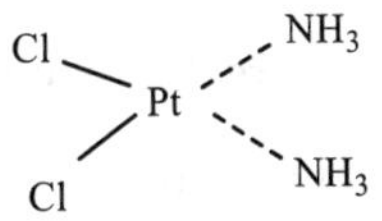

cis - Diammine dichloroplatinum

It is a platinum complex containing two ammonia molecule and two chlorine atom in *cis* configuration.

Mechanism of action: It acts by binding to DNA and interfering with its repair mechanism, eventually leading to cell death.

Use: It is used metastatic testicular tumor, metastatic ovarian tumors and advanced bladder cancer.

Chapter 3

ANTIANGINAL AGENTS

1. INTRODUCTION

The word angina (meaning in Greek: to choke) is used to describe the pain or discomfort of cardiac origin, which results in temporary ischemia of the myocardium, that is flow of blood is inadequate to maintain the metabolic demand of heart for oxygen and nutrients.

The coronary circulation supplies blood to the myocardial tissue to maintain cardiac function. It dilates the blood vessel to provide sufficient oxygen and other nutrient and to remove metabolites. Angina is caused by the coronary vessel constriction which prevents this blood flow.

Antianginal agents may improve angina by reducing the demand or by increasing the supply of oxygen and dilates coronary arteries and decrease after load.

2. CLASSIFICATION

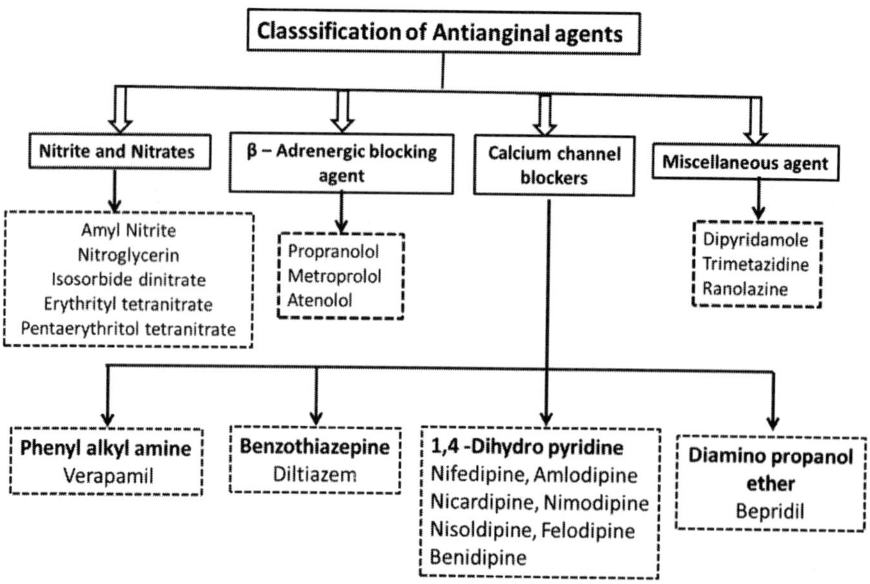

2.1 Nitrite and Nitrates

Organic nitrates are nitric acid esters of monohydric and polyhydric alcohols. They act as prodrugs for nitric oxide and must undergo enzymatic denitrification to mediate their pharmacodynamic effects. Important examples of organic nitrates are Amyl nitrite, Nitroglycerine, Isosorbide dinitrate, Erythrityl tetranitrate and Pentaerythritol tetranitrate. They are used to treat or prevent acute attacks of angina pectoris.

Mechanism of action: Organic nitrates, acts as a donor of nitric oxide (NO). They do not directly release NO; however, their nitrate groups interact with enzymes and intracellular sulfhydryl groups that which reduce the nitrate groups to NO or to S-nitrosothiol and then it is reduced to NO. The NO causes a relaxation of vascular smooth muscle via the stimulation of *guanylyl cyclase* and the subsequent increase of intracellular cyclic guanosine monophosphate (cGMP) concentration. A cGMP-dependent protein kinase promotes dephosphorylation of the light chain of myosin and the lowering reduction of Ca^{++} level. This leads to relaxation of smooth muscle tone. Arteriolar relaxation reduces systemic vascular resistance and systolic blood pressure decreasing cardiac afterload. Nitrates also cause increase in coronary blood flow. These combined effects decrease myocardial oxygen demand and relieves ischemia.

A. Amyl nitrite

$$(CH_3)_2.CH.CH_2.CH_2.O.NO$$

Isopentyl nitrite

It is a mixture of isomers containing not less than 97.0% and not more than 100.0% of $C_5H_{11}NO_2$.

Use: It is used to treat angina pectoris and to treat cyanide poisoning. It is also used as an antihypertensive agent.

B. Nitroglycerin (Myovin, Angised)

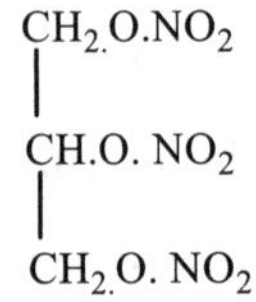

1, 2, 3 - Propanetriol trinitrate

Synthesis

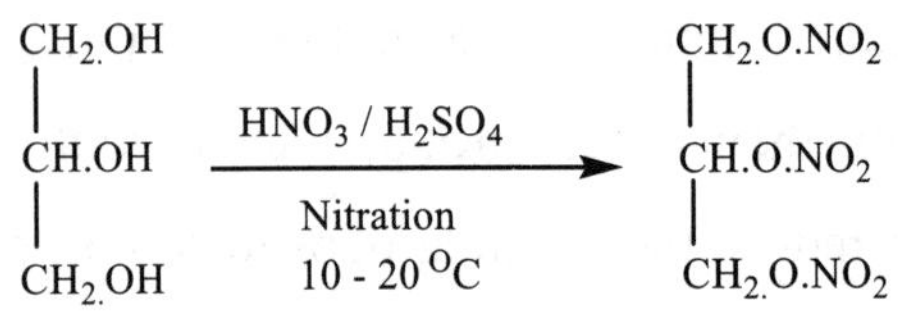

Glycerol   Nitroglycerin

Use: It is used as vasodilating agent. It is extensively used as an explosive in dynamite.

C. Pentaerythritol tetranitrate (Cardilate)

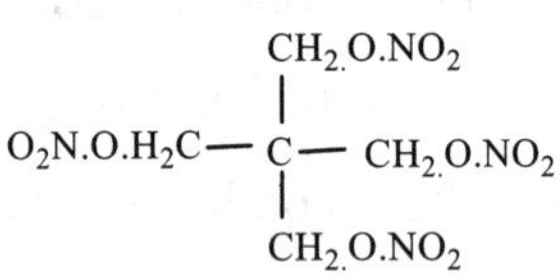

2, 2 - Bis (hydroxy methyl) - 1, 3 - propanediol tetranitrate

Use: It is used for the treatment of angina pectoris.

D. Isosorbide dinitrate (Isordil, Sorbitrate)

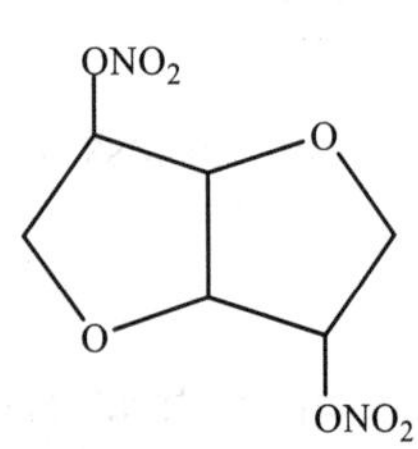

1, 4: 3, 6 - Dianhydro - D - glucitol dinitrate

Synthesis

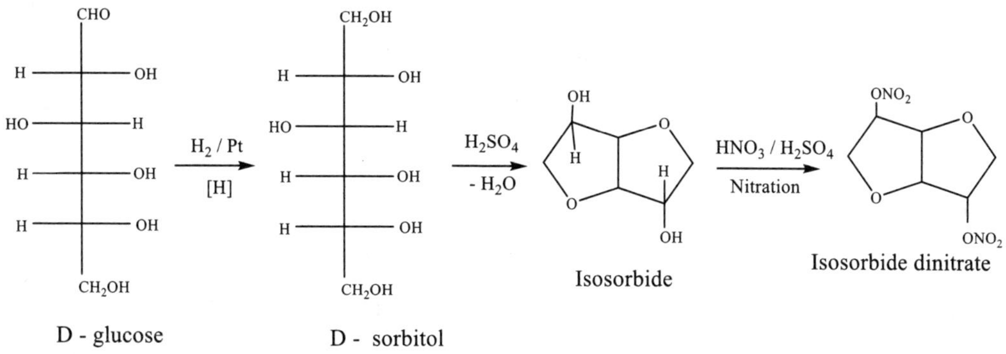

Use: It is effective in the treatment of acute angina attack.

2.2. Calcium Channel Blockers

Calcium channel blockers (CCB's) or calcium channel antagonists are drugs that block the entry of calcium into the muscle cells of the heart and arteries. They are divided into four classes based on their structure as Dihydropyridines (Nifedipine, Amlodipine), Phenylalkylamines (Verapamil), Benzothiazepines (Diltiazem) and Diamino propanol ether (Bepridil)

Mechanism of action: Calcium channel antagonists block the inward movement of calcium by binding to the L-type calcium channels in the heart and in smooth muscle of the peripheral vasculature. CCB's dilate coronary arteries and peripheral arterioles, but not veins. They also decrease cardiac contractility (negative inotropic effect) automaticity at the SA node and conduction at the AV node. Dilation of the coronary arteries increases myocardial oxygen supply.

a) Hypertension

Calcium channel antagonist's effectiveness in the treatment of hypertension is related to a decrease in peripheral resistance accompanied by increases in cardiac index.

b) Angina pectoris

Calcium channel blockers act as coronary vasodilators, producing variable and dose-dependent reductions in myocardial oxygen demand, contractility and arterial pressure. These combined pharmacologic effects are advantageous and make these agents as effective as β-blockers in the treatment of angina pectoris.

c) Arrhythmias

Calcium channel blockers act as antiarrhythmic based on their depressant action at the SA and AV nodes. Their ability to inhibit the AV node is employed in the management of supraventricular tachyarrhythmias, such as: atrial fibrillation, atrial flutter and paroxysmal supraventricular tachycardia.

There are two major categories of calcium channel antagonists based on their primary physiologic effects are dihydropyridines and non-dihydropyridines.

The non-dihydropyridines (Verapamil and Diltiazem) have inhibitory effects on the sinoatrial (SA) and atrioventricular (AV) nodes are resulting in a slowing of cardiac conduction and contractility. They also decrease heart rate. This allows for the treatment of hypertension, reduces oxygen demand and helps to control the rate in tachydysrhythmias.
The dihydropyridines, in therapeutic dosing, have a little direct effect on the myocardium, and more peripheral vasodilators so they are used for hypertension, post-intracranial hemorrhage associated vasospasm and migraines.

2.2.1 1, 4 - Dihydro pyridine

Dihydropyridines (DHP) all end in "**PINE**". DHP drugs are inhibitors of L-type calcium-dependent calcium channels that are mainly used as antihypertensive. All these compounds are 4- substituted phenyl-1,4-dhydropyridine derivatives and are photosensitive.

Mechanism of action: 1, 4-Dihydro pyridines are peripheral arterial vasodilator which acts directly on vascular smooth muscle. The binding of DHP to voltage-dependent L-type calcium channels and possibly receptor-operated channels in vascular smooth muscle results in an inhibition of calcium influx through these channels. The reduction in calcium influx causes arterial vasodilation and decreased peripheral vascular resistance which results in reduced arterial blood pressure.

Table 3.1 Structural feature is important for activity

<table>
<tr>
<td>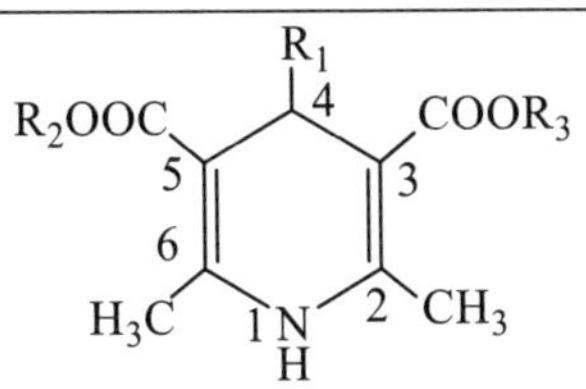</td>
<td>

- 1, 4 - Dihydro pyridine ring is essential for activity.
- A phenyl ring substitution at 4th position optimizes activity.
- The 3rd and 5th position ester group optimizes activity. Any other electron withdrawing substitution results in agonist activity.
- When the ester at C_3 and C_5 are non-identical the C_4 become chiral and stereo selectivity is observed. S-enantiomers have proved to be more effective.

</td>
</tr>
</table>

Table 3.2 Structure of 1, 4 – Dihydro Pyridine Derivatives

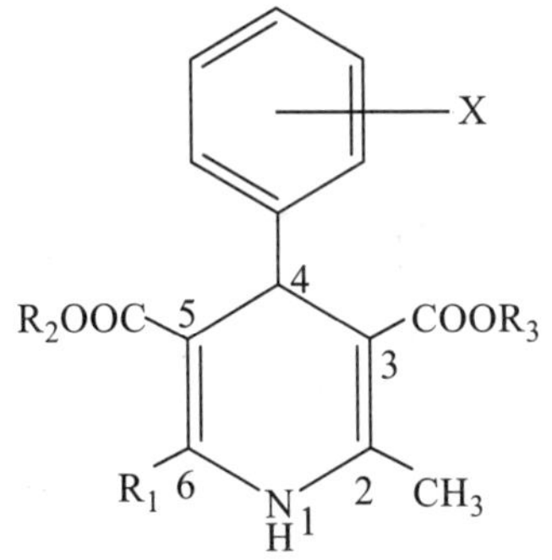

S. No	Compounds	R_1	R_2	R_3	X
1.	Amlodipine	$-CH_2O(CH_2)_2NH_2$	$-C_2H_5$	$-CH_3$	2 - Cl
2.	Felodipine	$-CH_3$	$-C_2H_5$	$-CH_3$	2, 3 – dichloro
3.	Nifedipine	$-CH_3$	$-CH_3$	$-CH_3$	2 - NO_2
4.	Nicardipine	$-CH_3$	$C_6H_5.CH_2.N(CH_3).(CH_2)_2.-$	$-CH_3$	3 - NO_2
5.	Nimodipine	$-CH_3$	$-CH_2CH_2OCH_3$	$-CH(CH_3)_2$	3 - NO_2

A. Amlodipine (Amlibon, Stamlo)

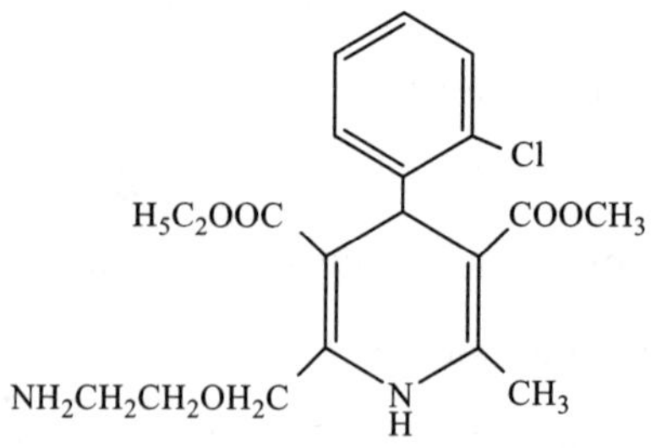

(RS) - 3 - Ethyl - 5 - methyl - 2 - [(2 - Amino ethoxy) methyl] - 4 - (2 - chloro phenyl) - 6 - methyl - 1, 4 - dihydropyridine - 3, 5 - dicarboxylate

Use: It is used as antianginal and antihypertensive agent.

B. Nifedipine (Nebicard, Angiblock)

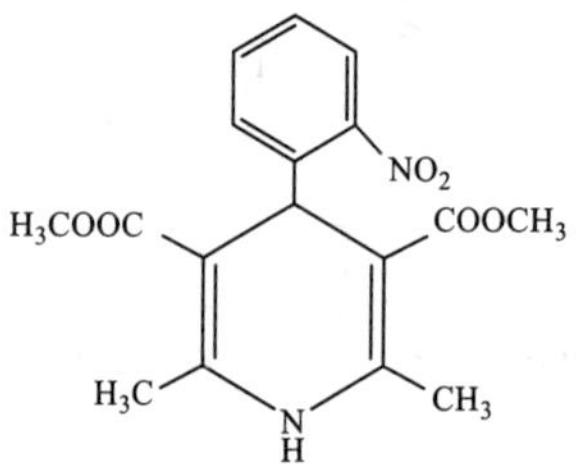

3, 5 - Dimethyl - 2, 6 - dimethyl - 4 - (2 - nitro phenyl) - 1, 4 - dihydro pyridine - 3, 5 - dicarboxylate

Use: It is used in the treatment of vasospastic angina and hypertension.

C. Nimodipine (Nimotop)

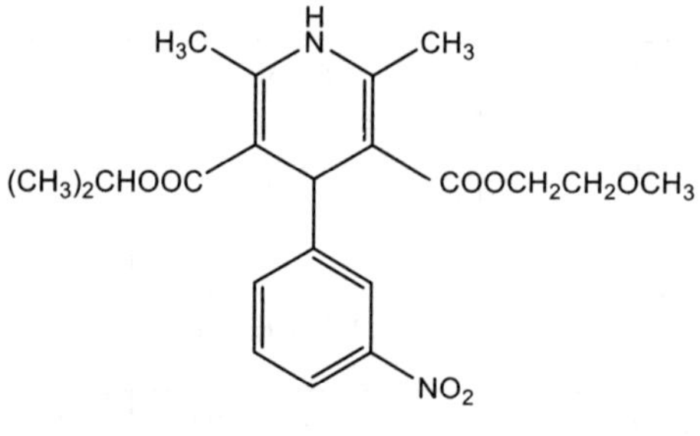

3 - (2 - Methoxyethyl) - 5 - propan - 2 - yl - 2,6 - dimethyl - 4 - (3 - nitrophenyl) - 1,4 - dihydropyridine - 3,5 - dicarboxylate

Use: It is mainly used in the prevention of cerebral vasospasm and resultant ischemia.

D. Felodipine (Felogard, Plendil)

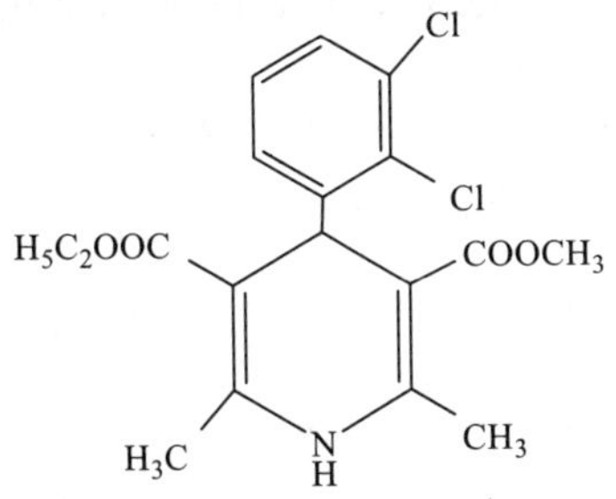

3, 5 - Dimethyl - 2, 6 - dimethyl - 4 - (2, 3 - dichloro phenyl) - 1, 4 - dihydropyridine - 3, 5 - pyridine dicarboxylate

Use: It is used in the treatment of angina and essential hypertension.

E. Nicardipine (Cardene)

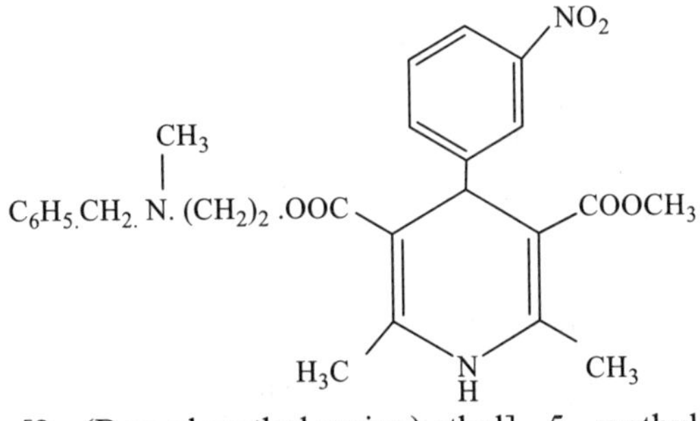

3 - [2 - (Benzyl methyl amino) ethyl] - 5 - methyl - 2, 6 - dimethyl - 4 - (3 - nitro phenyl) - 1, 4 - dihydropyridine - 3, 5 - dicarboxylate

Use: It is a more potent vasodilator of the systemic, coronary, cerebral and renal vasculature. It is used to treat hypertension and angina.

2.2.2 Phenyl Alkylamine

A. Verapamil (Calaptin, Vasopten)

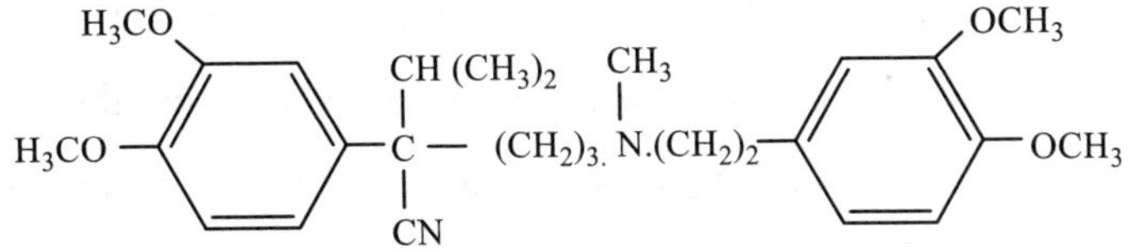

5 - (3, 4 - Dimethoxy phenethyl) methyl amino] - 2 - (3, 4 - dimethoxy phenyl) - 2 - isopropyl pentyl nitrile

The R-enantiomer is more effective in reducing the blood pressure whereas the S-enantiomer 20 times more potent than the R-enantiomer as antiarrhythmic.

Mechanism of action: Verapamil is an L-type calcium channel blocker that also has antiarrhythmic activity. Specifically, its effect on L-type calcium channels in the heart causes a reduction in inotropy and chronotropy, thus reducing heart rate and blood pressure.

Use: It is used in the treatment of angina pectoris, arrhythmias from ischemic myocardial syndromes and supraventricular arrhythmias.

2.2.3 Benzothiazepine

A. Diltiazem hydrochloride (Dilgard)

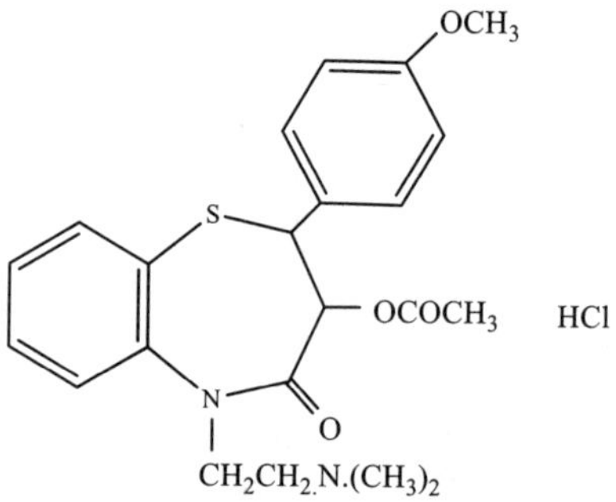

(+) - Cis - 3 - (acetyloxy) - 5 - [(2 - dimethyl amino) ethyl] - 2, 3 - dihydro - 2 - (4 - methoxy phenyl) - 1, 5 - benzothiazepin - 4 - (5H) - one hydrochloride

Diltiazem has two chiral centers (C_2 and C_3), the *levo* rotatory *cis* antipode is more active form.

Mechanisms of action: It works by inhibiting the calcium influx into cardiac and vascular smooth muscle during depolarization. Compared to dihydropyridine drugs, that preferentially act on vascular smooth muscle and Verapamil that directly acts on the heart muscle, Diltiazem displays an intermediate specificity to target both the cardiac and vascular smooth muscle. They also have inhibitory effects on the sinoatrial (SA) and atrioventricular (AV) nodes resulting in slowing of cardiac conduction and contractility. They also decrease heart rate. This allows for the treatment of hypertension, angina, and helps to control the rate in tachydysrhythmias.

Use: It is used in the treatment of hypertension, angina pectoris and also used as antiarrhythmic agent.

2.2.4 Diamino Propanol Ethers

A. Bepridil (Vascor)

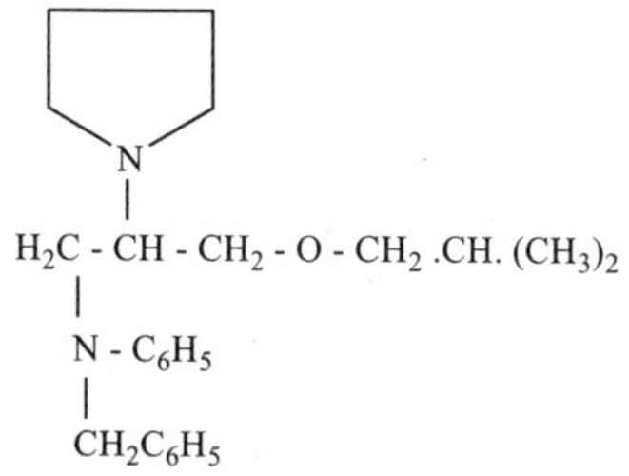

β - [(2 - Methyl propoxy) methyl] - N - phenyl - N - (phenyl methyl) - 1 - pyrrolidine ethyl amine

It is a second-generation alkyl amine type calcium channel blocker.

Mechanism of action: It possess inhibitory effects on both the slow L type calcium channel and fast sodium inward currents in myocardial and vascular smooth muscle, interferes with calcium binding to calmodulin, and blocks both voltage and receptor operated calcium channels. Bepridil inhibits the transmembrane influx of calcium ions into cardiac and vascular smooth muscle.

Use: It is used as vasodilator and antianginal agent.

2.3 Miscellaneous

A. Dipyridamole (Cardiwell, Persantin)

It is a p*hosphodiesterase*-3-inhibitor causes a long acting and selective coronary vasodilator by increasing coronary blood flow via selective dilation of the coronary arteries.

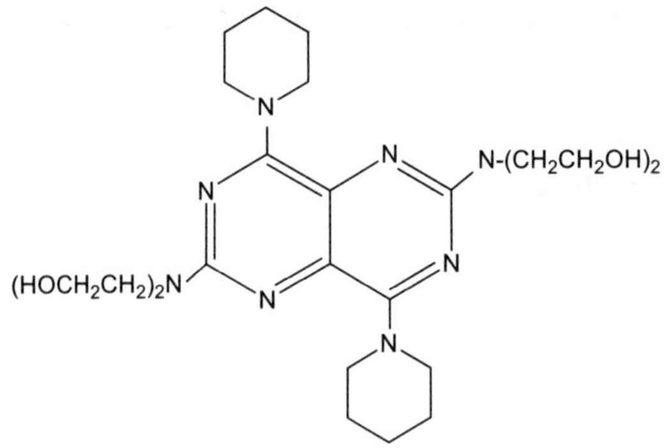

2, 2 - Bis [diethanol amino] - 4, 8 -
dipiperidino pyrimido - [5,4 - d] - pyrimidine

Mechanism of action: It inhibits *adenosine deaminase* in erythrocytes and interferes with the uptake of vasodilator adenosine by erythrocytes. These actions potentiate the effect of prostacyclin which acts as an inhibitor to platelet aggregation.

Use: It is a long acting vasodilator. Its vasodilating effect is selective for the coronary system. It is used to treat angina pectoris.

Chapter 4

DIURETICS

1. INTRODUCTION

Diuretics are drugs that promote the output of urine excreted by Kidneys. The primary action of most of the diuretics are the direct inhibition of Na^+ transport at one or more of the four major anatomical sites along the nephron, where Na^+ reabsorption takes place. The increased excretion of water and electrolytes by the kidneys is dependent on three different processes viz., glomerular filtration, tubular reabsorption (active and passive) and tubular secretion.

Diuretics are very effective in the treatment of cardiac edema, specifically the one related with congestive heart failure. They are employed extensively in various types of disorders, for example, nephritic syndrome, diabetes insipidus, nutritional edema, cirrhosis of the liver, hypertension, edema of pregnancy and also to lower intraocular and cerebrospinal fluid pressure.

1.1 Mechanism of action of Diuretics

Diuretic drugs increase urine output by the kidney. If the kidney excretes more sodium, then water excretion will also increase. Most diuretics produce diuresis by inhibiting the reabsorption of sodium at different segments of the renal tubular system. Sometimes a combination of two diuretics is given because this can be significantly more effective than either compound alone (synergistic effect). The reason for this is that, one nephron segment can compensate for altered sodium reabsorption at another nephron segment; therefore, blocking multiple nephron sites significantly enhances efficacy. Reduced reabsorption of sodium results in increased urinary loss of both sodium and water, leading to a reduction in plasma volume and a reduction of blood pressure.

1.2 Therapeutic Uses of Diuretics

- **Congestive heart failure**: Furosemide, Sodium Ethacrynate, Hydrochlorothiazide or Chlorthalidone may be used.
- **Essential hypertension**: The thiazides usually serve as primary antihypertensive
- **Hepatic cirrhosis**: Potassium-sparing diuretics like Spironolactone may be employed
- **Nephrotic syndrome**: Dietary sodium restriction may be combined with a thiazide diuretic, adding Spironolactone to control secondary hyperaldosteronism.
- **Chronic renal failure**: Careful attention to salt and water balance is required. A Loop diuretic like Furosemide may be useful in controlling both edema and hypertension.
- **Edema**: Osmotic diuretic Mannitol may be employed
- **Glaucoma:** The *Carbonic anhydrase* inhibitors (Acetazolamide) may be use in the long-term treatment of primary open-angle glaucoma.
- **Intraocular surgery**: The osmotic diuretic (Glycerol, Mannitol) are used to reduce intraocular pressure in ocular surgical procedures.
- **Diabetes insipidus**: The thiazides exhibit paradoxical antidiuretic action in patients with diabetes insipidus.

2. CLASSIFICATION

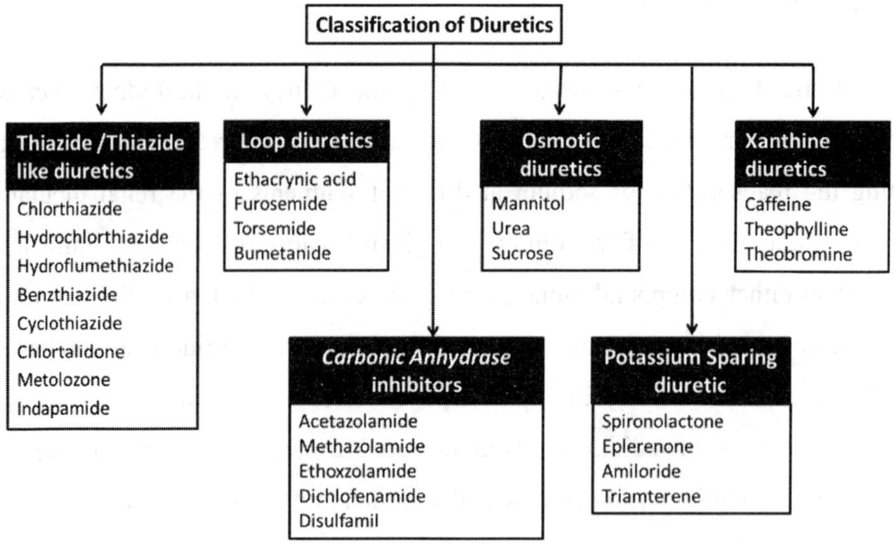

2.1 *Carbonic anhydrase* Inhibitors

This class of diuretics inhibits *carbonic anhydrase* in the membrane and cytoplasm of the epithelial cells. They are derived from sulphonamide antibacterial. Two groups of *carbonic anhydrase* inhibitors are

- ✓ Heterocyclic sulphonamide eg. Acetazolamide, Methazolamide
- ✓ *m*-disulfamoyl benzene derivatives eg. Dichlorphenamide

Mechanism of action: The primary site of action is in proximal tubules. It works to reabsorb sodium, bicarbonate and chloride. Once the *carbonic anhydrase* is inhibited, sodium, bicarbonate and chloride get excreted rather than reabsorbed; this also leads to the excretion of excess water.

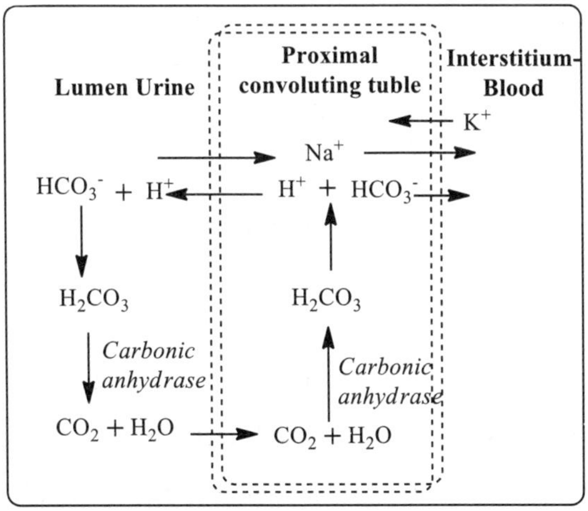

Fig. 4.1 Mechanism of *Carbonic anhydrase*

Carbonic anhydrase catalyses the reaction of CO_2 and H_2O leading to H_2CO_3 which spontaneously ionizes to H^+ and HCO_3^- (Fig. 4.1). In the proximal tubule, Na^+-H^+ antiport in the epithelial cells transports H^+ into tubular lumen in exchange for Na^+ movement into it. Na^+ in the cytoplasm is pumped out to the interstitium by sodium pump.

H^+ in the lumen reacts with HCO_3^- to form H_2CO_3. H_2CO_3 is dehydrated to CO_2 and H_2O. This reaction is catalyzed by *carbonic anhydrase* in the luminal membrane.

Both CO_2 and H_2O can permeate into cells and rehydrate to form H_2CO_3. The rehydration is catalyzed by the cytoplasmic *carbonic anhydrase* H_2CO_3 dissociates to form H^+ which is secreted into lumen and HCO_3- which is transported into interstitium. Inhibition of anhydrase thus inhibits HCO_3^- reabsorption. Accumulation of HCO_3^- in the tubular lumen subsequently inhibits Na^+, H^+ exchange and Na^+ reabsorption.

The increase in Na^+ concentration in the tubular fluid may be compensated partially by increased NaCl reabsorption in later segments of the tubule. Thus, the diuretic effect of the *carbonic anhydrase* inhibitor is mild. These are the weakest of the diuretics and seldom used in cardiovascular disease. Their main use is in the treatment of glaucoma.

A. Acetazolamide (Diamox)

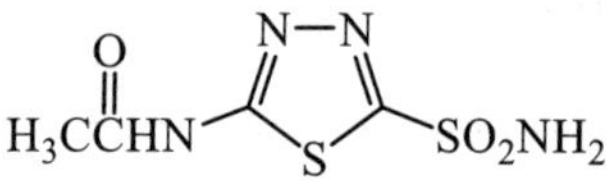

N - [5 -(Aminosulfonyl) -
1, 3, 4 - thiadiazol - 2 - yl]
acetamide

It is proto type *carbonic anhydrase* inhibitors. These agents decrease the activity of *carbonic anhydrase* at other sites in the body like CNS, eye, lungs and gastrointestinal tract. *Carbonic anhydrase* inhibitors are used in the treatment of glaucoma, edema and epileptic.

Synthesis

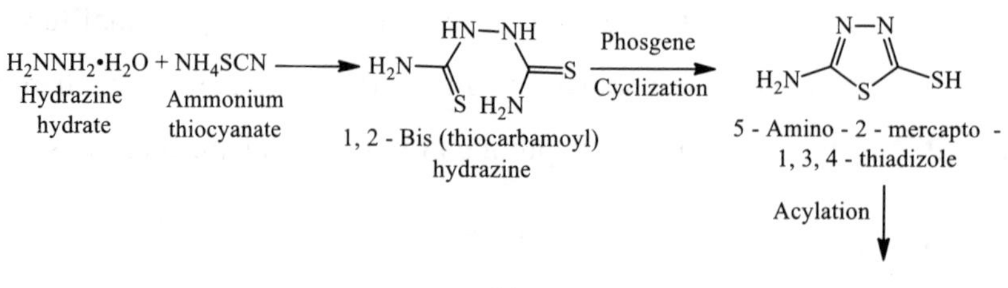

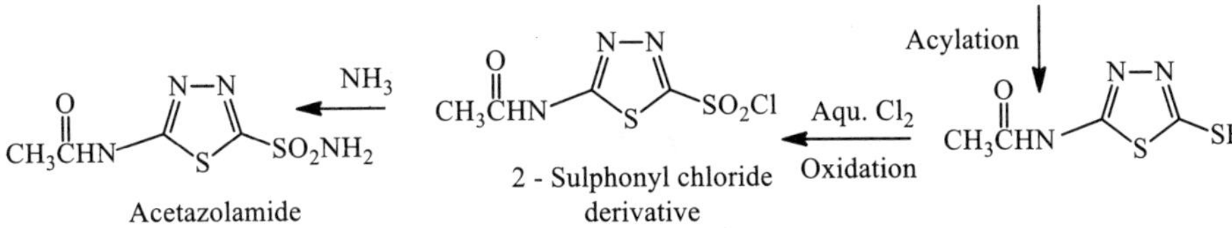

Mechanism of action: It is a *carbonic anhydrase* inhibitor and the diuretic action depends upon the accumulation of HCO_3^- in the tubular lumen subsequently inhibits Na^+, H^+ exchange and Na^+ reabsorption. This leads to the excretion of excess water, lowering blood pressure, intracranial pressure and intraocular pressure. In eye, it causes a reduction in aqueous humour and so used in the treatment of glaucoma. The anticonvulsant activity of Acetazolamide may depend on a direct inhibition of *carbonic anhydrase* in the CNS, which decreases carbon dioxide tension in the pulmonary alveoli, thus increasing arterial oxygen tension.

Use: It is employed in the treatment of drug-induced edema and edema caused by congestive heart failure, petit mal epilepsy and menstrual related epilepsy. There are use is in the treatment of glaucoma, idiopathic intracranial hypertension and altitude sickness.

B. Methazolamide (Neptazane)

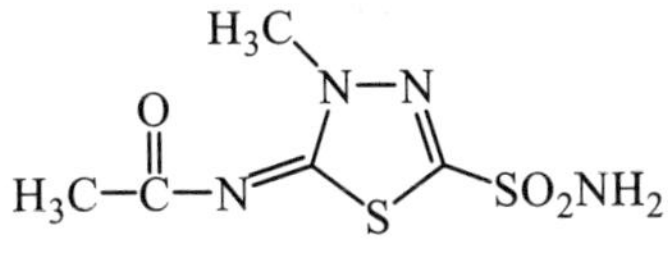

N - [5 - (Aminosulfonyl) - 3 - methyl - 1, 3, 4 - thiadiazol - 2 (3H) - ylidene] acetamide

It is topical *carbonic anhydrase* inhibitor

Mechanism of action: It is a potent inhibitor of *carbonic anhydrase*.

Use: It is employed in the treatment of drug-induced oedema, caused by congestive heart failure, petit mal epilepsy and menstrual related epilepsy.

C. Dichlorphenamide (Daranide)

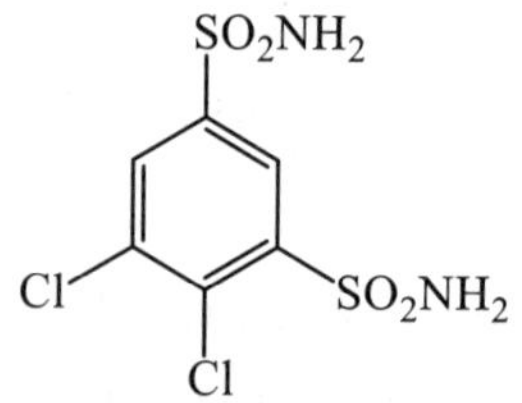

4,5 - Dichloro - m - benzene disulphonamide

It is benzene -1, 3 - disulfonamide derivative

Mechanism of action: It is a *carbonic anhydrase* inhibitor; it partially suppresses the secretion of aqueous humor in the eye and so reduces intraocular pressure.

Use: It is used for the treatment of both primary and secondary glaucoma.

2.2 Thiazide/Thiazide like Diuretics

Thiazide (benzothiadiazine) diuretics were originally developed more than 50 years ago as a result of chemical modification of Sulfanilamide. Chlorothiazide was the first thiazide, marketed, in the year 1957. This class of drugs refers to both sulphonamide containing compounds as well as benzothiadiazine ring. The term "thiazide" is also often used for drugs with a similar action that do not have the thiazide chemical structure, such as Chlorthalidone and Metolazone. Sometimes they are called low ceiling diuretics because increasing the dose above therapeutic doses does not make any change in diuretic activity. Thiazide diuretics are mainly used to treat hypertension and edema

Thiazides have the following general chemical structure

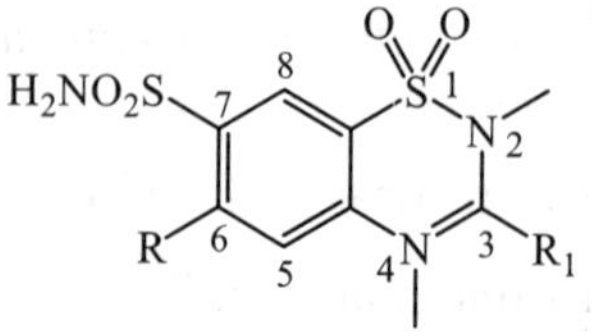

Hydrogen atom at 2nd position is more acidic, due to the presence of neighboring electron withdrawing sulfone group. These acidic protons make salt with sodium used for intravenous administration.

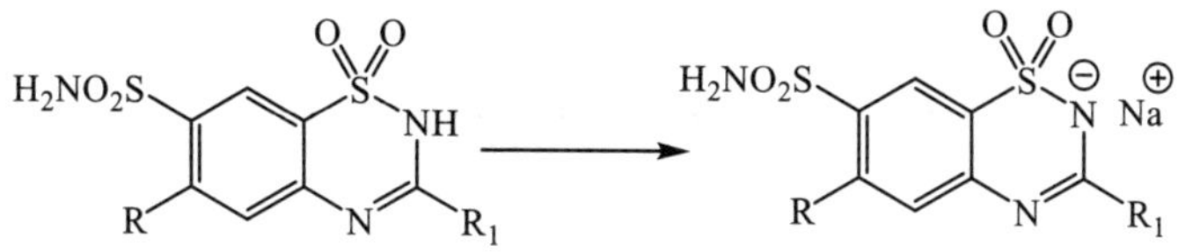

Saturation of the double bond between 3rd and 4th position increases the potency, approximately 3 to 10-fold. For example, Hydrochlorthiazide is found to be 10 times more active than Chlorothiazide and have lower toxicity. A free sulfamoyl group at 7th position is essential for activity.

Mechanism of action: They are the most commonly used diuretic; inhibit the sodium-chloride transporter in the distal tubule. Thiazides decrease sodium reabsorption which increases fluid loss in urine, which in turn decreases extracellular fluid and plasma volume. This reduces cardiac output and lowers blood pressure. They also cause an increase in the excretion of Cl^-, K^+ and HCO_3^- ions.

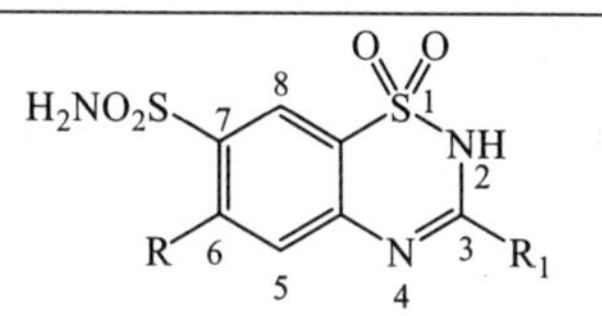 Thiazide Diuretics	**Generic Name**	**R**	**R_1**
	Chlorthiazide	- Cl	- H

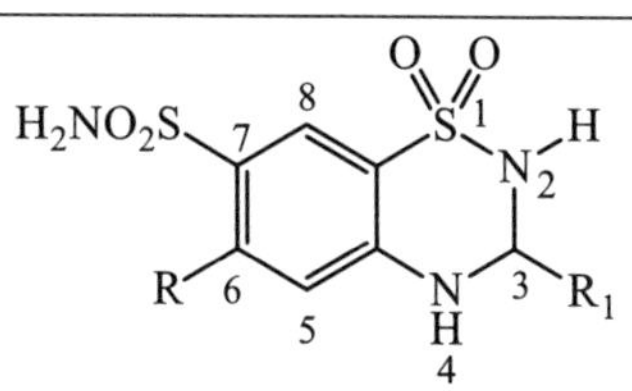 Hydrothiazide Diuretics	**Generic Name**	**R**	**R_1**
	Hydrochlorothiazide	- Cl	- H
	Hydroflumethiazide	- CF_3	- H
	Cyclothiazide	- Cl	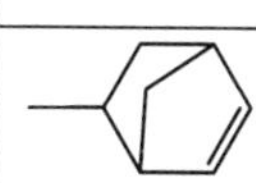

A. Chlorothiazide (Diuril)

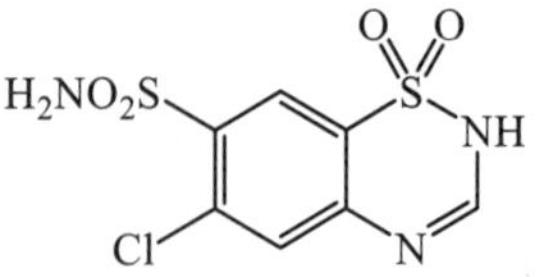

6 - Chloro - 2H - 1, 2, 4 - benzothiadiazine - 7 - sulphonamide - 1, 1 - dioxide

Synthesis

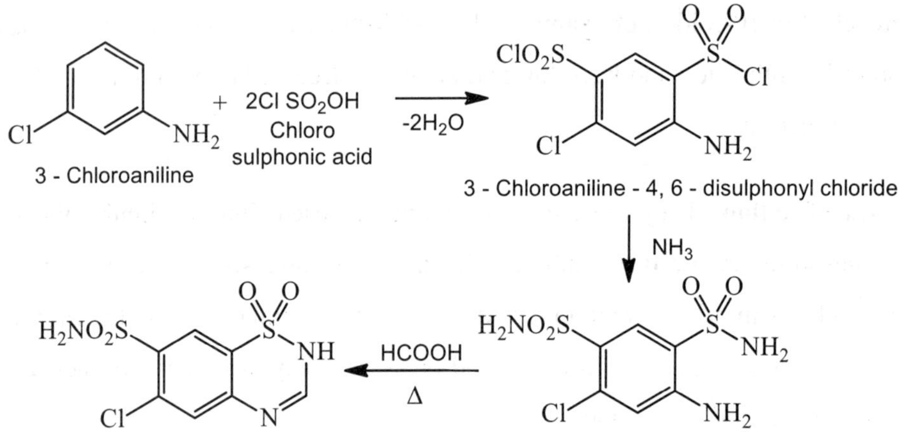

Use: It is used in the treatment of edema associated with congestive heart failure, hypertension and renal and hepatic disorders.

B. Hydrochlorthiazide (Hydride)

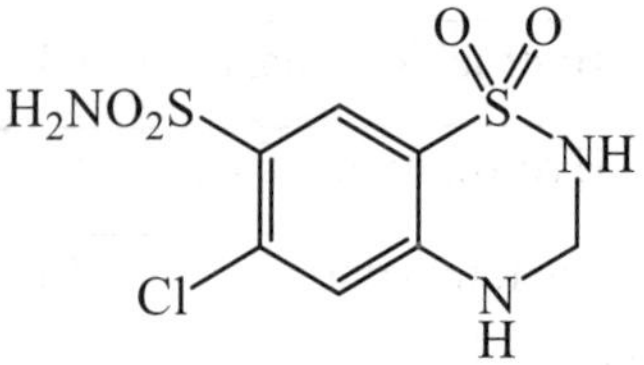

6 - Chloro - 3, 4 - dihydro - 2H - 1, 2, 4 - benzothiadiazine - 7 - sulphonamide - 1,1 - dioxide

Use: It is used in the treatment of edema associated with congestive heart failure and renal and hepatic disorders. It is 10 times more potent than other thiazide diuretics.

C. Hydroflumethiazide (Saluron)

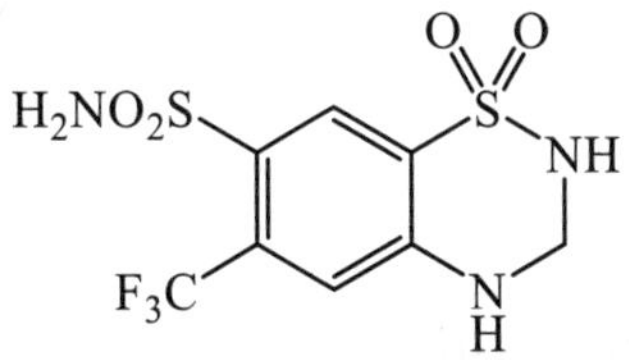

3, 4 - Dihydro - 6 - (trifluoromethyl) - 2H - 1, 2, 4 - benzothiadiazine - 7 - sulphonamide - 1,1 - dioxide

Use: It is a potent diuretic used in the management of edema associated with cardiac failure, premenstrual tension and hepatic cirrhosis.

D. Cyclothiazide (Doburil)

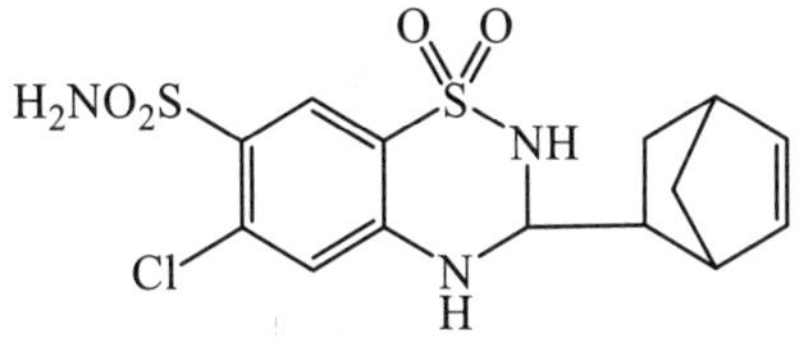

6 - Chloro - 3, 4 - dihydro - 3 - (5 - norbornen - 2 - yl) - 2H - 1, 2, 4 - benzothiadiazine - 7 - sulphonamide - 1,1 - dioxide

Use: It has diuretic and antihypertensive properties.

2.3 High Ceiling or Loop Diuretics

Loop diuretics, also known as high ceiling or high efficacy diuretics, are important drugs for the treatment of several disorders. They have a higher capacity for diuresis compared to other diuretics because they act at the level of the thick ascending limb of the Loop of Henle, where 20–25% of the sodium that is filtered through the glomerulus is reabsorbed. They are used to treat hypertension and edema often due to congestive heart failure, liver failure or chronic kidney disease.

Mechanism of action: Loop diuretics promote diuresis by blocking tubular reabsorption of sodium and chloride in the proximal and distal tubules, as well as in the thick ascending Loop of Henle. This is achieved through competitive inhibition of sodium-potassium-chloride co-transporters in the nephron, resulting in excretion of water along with sodium, chloride, magnesium and calcium.

A. Bumetanide (Bumex)

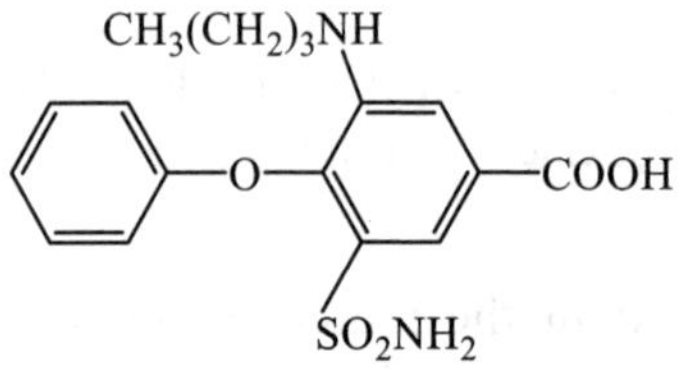

3 - Butylamino - 4 - phenoxy - 5 - sulphamoyl benzoic acid

Use: It is used in the treatment of edema associated with congestive heart failure, hepatic and renal disease including the nephrotic syndrome.

B. Furosemide (Lasix)

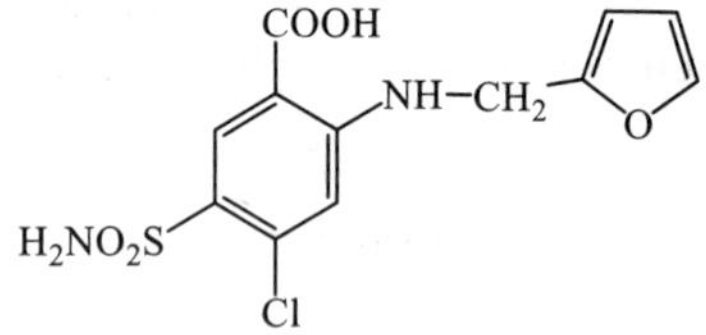

4 - Chloro - N - furfuryl - 5 - sulphamoyl anthranilic acid

Synthesis

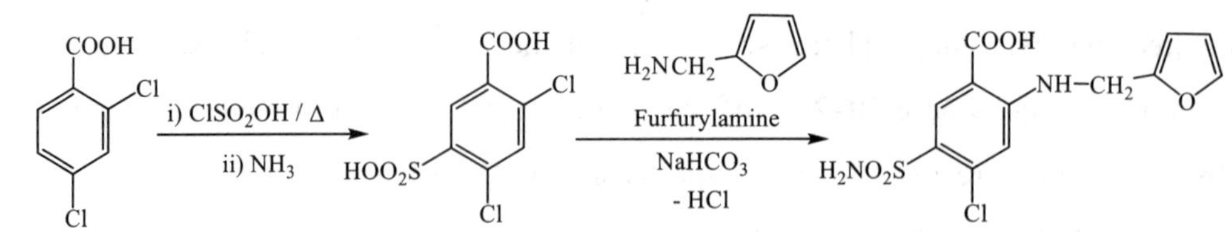

2,4 - Dichloro benzoic acid

Furosemide

Use: It is used for the treatment of oedema associated with renal disease, nephritic syndrome, cirrhosis of liver and congestive heart failure.

C. Ethacrynic acid (Edecrin)

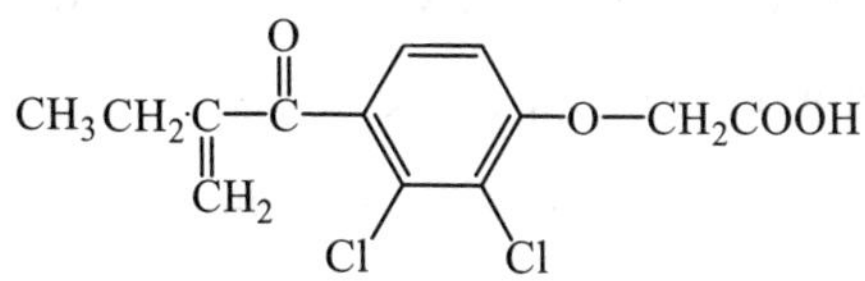

2, 3 - Dichloro - 4 - (2 - methylene butyryl) phenoxyacetic acid

Use: It is a high ceiling diuretic used in the treatment of congestive heart failure, cirrhosis of the liver, renal disease and the nephritic syndrome.

2.4 Potassium Sparing Diuretics

Potassium-sparing diuretics are diuretics that result in increased urine production and also lower blood pressure while increasing serum levels of potassium. The potassium-sparing diuretics are Spironolactone, Triamterene and Amiloride, They are called K^+-sparing diuretics because they do not produce hypokalemia like Loop and thiazide diuretics. Their major use is in conjunction with the thiazides or Loop diuretics. Such a combined therapy reduces potassium loss, minimizes alkalosis and is sometimes effective in refractory oedema.

A. Spironolactone (Aldactone)

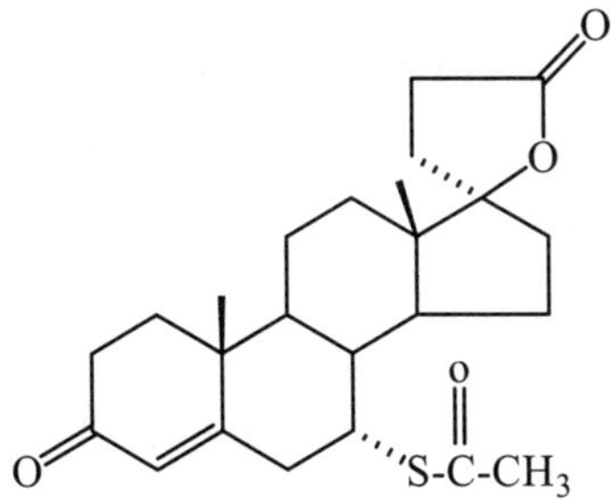

7α - Acetyl thio - 17α - hydroxy - 3 - oxo - pregn - 4 - en - 21 - carboxylic acid - γ - lactone

It is structurally similar to progesterone and as a result is associated with progestogenic and antiandrogenic effects.

Mechanism of action: It antagonizes the actions of aldosterone (aldosterone receptor antagonists) at the distal segment of the distal tubule. Normally, aldosterone binds to the mineralocorticoid receptor and enhances the activity of epithelial sodium channels and Na^+/K^+-*ATPase* pump. Therefore, by blocking the mineralocorticoid receptor, aldosterone antagonists inhibit the activity of epithelial sodium channel and the Na^+/K^+-ATPase pump, reducing Na^+ reabsorption and producing mild natriuresis and diuresis. Inhibiting the basolateral Na^+/K^+-*ATPase* pump reduces the excretion of K^+, increasing the amount of K^+ in blood.

Use: It is useful in cirrhosis of liver, aldosterone-secreting tumors and high-renin hypertension.

B. Amiloride (Biduret)

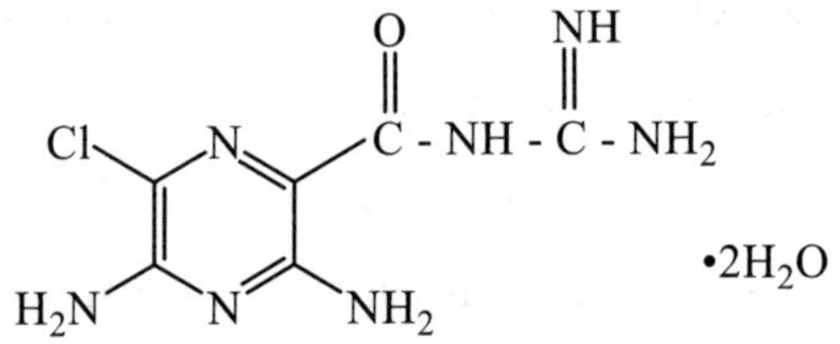

3, 5 - Diamino - N - (amino imino methyl) -
6 - chloro pyrazine carboxamide

It is an antikaliuretic diuretic agent and is a pyrazinoyl-guanidine derivative

Mechanism of action: It is not an aldosterone antagonist. It inhibits epithelial sodium channel on the luminal membrane, preventing Na^+ moving from the tubular lumen into the cell. This keeps Na^+ in the lumen of the tubule, therefore facilitating natriuresis. Reduced entry of Na^+ into the cell also reduces the amount of Na^+ that can be exchanged for K^+ at the *ATPase* pump. The Na^+/K^+-*ATPase* pump unable to exchange Na^+ for K^+, the K^+ stays in the blood stream. Compared with thiazides and Loop diuretics, Amiloride is therefore potassium sparing diuretics.

Use: It is used adjunctively with thiazides and Loop diuretics for the treatment of chronic heart failure or uncomplicated essential hypertension.

C. Triamterene (Ditide)

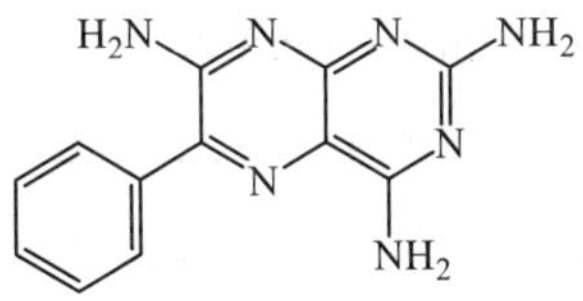

2, 4, 7 - Triamino - 6 - phenyl pteridine

It is a potassium sparing diuretic with substituted pteridine ring

Mechanism of action: It inhibit epithelial sodium channel on the luminal membrane, preventing Na^+ moving from the tubular lumen into the cell. This keeps Na^+ in the lumen of the tubule, therefore facilitating natriuresis. Reduced entry of Na^+ into the cell also reduces the amount of Na^+ that can be exchanged for K^+ at the ATPase pump. The Na^+/ K^+-*ATPase* pump unable to exchange Na^+ for K^+, the K^+ stays in the bloodstream.

Use: It is used in the treatment of edema associated with nephritic syndrome, cirrhosis of liver and congestive heart failure.

2.5 Osmotic Diuretics

Osmotic diuretics are agents that inhibit the reabsorption of solute and water by altering osmotic driving forces along the nephron. Unlike the other classes of diuretics, osmotic diuretics do not inhibit a specific membrane transport protein; they simply affect water transport across the cells of the nephron through the generation of an osmotic pressure gradient.

A. Mannitol (Osmitrol)

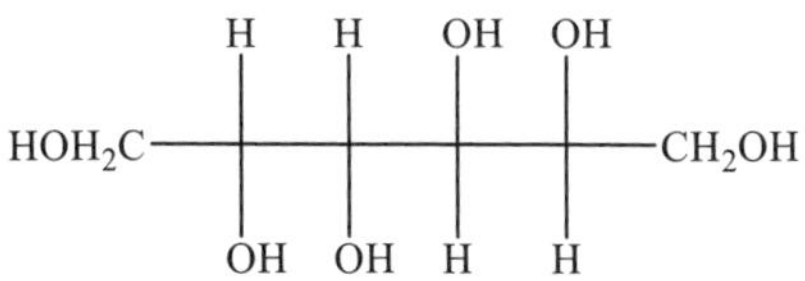

Hexan - 1, 2, 3, 4, 5, 6 - hexol

It is a polysaccharide diuretic, an isomer of sorbitol. It is given intravenously and freely eliminated by glomerular filtration.

Mechanism of action: Osmotic diuretics significantly increase the osmolarity of plasma and tubular fluid. The osmotic force thus generated prevents water reabsorption and also extracts water from the intracellular compartment, expands extracellular fluid volume and increases renal blood flow resulting in reduced medulla tonicity. The primary site of action for osmotic diuretics is the Loop of Henle and the proximal tubule where the membrane is most permeable to water

Use: Commonly used as diuretic and to treat or prevent medical conditions that caused by an increase in body fluids/water (eg. cerebral edema, glaucoma, kidney failure).

Chapter

ANTIHYPERTENSIVE AGENTS 5

1. INTRODUCTION

Hypertension is defined as a condition in which systolic and/or diastolic blood pressure exceeds above 140/90 mm Hg. It is not a single disease; it results from defects in hemodynamic and biochemical function in the body.

Agents that lower the blood pressure are called the antihypertensive agent. These drugs reduce the cardiac output or reduce the total peripheral resistance without correcting the cause.

Hypertension has been divided into two major divisions according to the etiology.

- Primary or Essential hypertension: Where definite cause is not known. This is the common form of hypertension.
- Secondary hypertension: Due to renal, endocrine and vascular disorder.

Many mechanisms operate in equilibrium with each other in order to maintain a constant blood pressure. These include central mechanism, peripheral adrenergic activity, baro-chemo receptor, cardiac output, viscosity of blood, renin-angiotensin-aldosterone system, vascular factor, blood volume etc.

The vascular fluctuation in the circulation are communicated and controlled by baro-chemo receptor. Baro receptor is pressure sensitive receptor located in the walls of heart and blood vessels. When there is a fall in blood pressure in carotid sinus, it stimulates the sympathetic nervous system and result in vasoconstriction (ie. increase in blood pressure). On the other hand, increase in the blood pressure activates the baro receptor, resulting in arterial dilatation thus opposing permanent hypertension. Loss of this inhibitor activity of baro receptor leads to hypertension. Chemo receptors located in vessel walls are sensitive to the oxygen content in blood. Both these receptors are mediated through the release of renin, which activates angiotensin - aldosterone system.

The various factors which lead to hypertension are

- Neural factor: Stress and emotionality cause excessive sympathetic outflow from the brain may result in increased cardiac output and elevated peripheral resistance.
- Renin-angiotensin system which can cause hypertension like blood vessel constriction, increased blood volume and increased cardiac output.
- The inability of the kidney to excrete an adequate daily amount of salt and water, result in increased blood volume.

2. CLASSIFICATION

Antihypertensive drugs are classified as

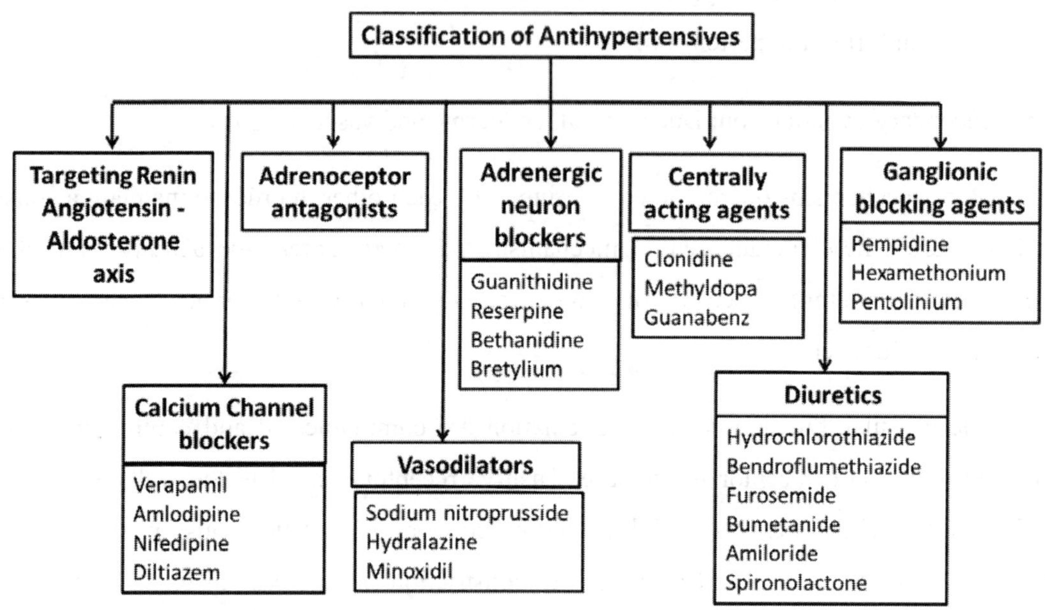

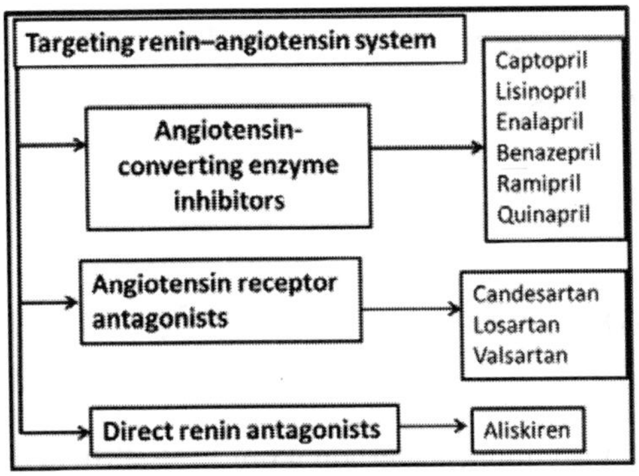

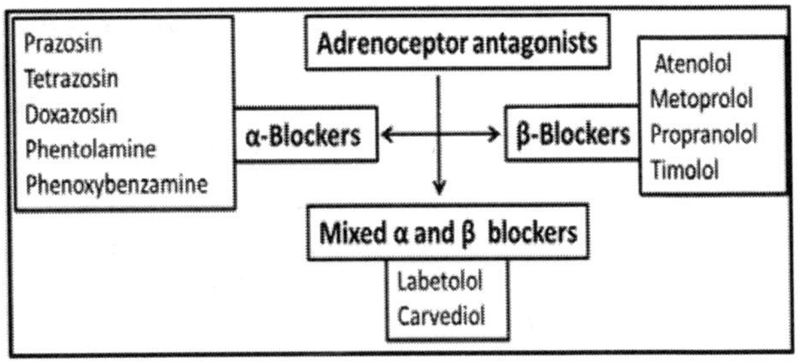

2.1 **Adreno Receptor Antagonist**

Adreno receptor blockers antagonize catecholamines at adrenergic receptors. These receptors are classified as β1, present mainly within the heart and kidneys and β2, present throughout the body in lungs, blood vessels and muscle. The first generation β-blockers are nonselective that they block both β_1 and β_2. The second generation β-blockers are cardio-selective that they are selective for β_1-adreneo receptor. The third generation β-blockers are mixed α_1/β_1-blockers. They are used as vasodilators. These drugs slow the heart rate and decrease the force of contraction. It is used in the treatment hypertension, coronary artery disease, arrhythmias and open angle glaucoma.

The reduction in arterial pressure achieved by β-blocker is attributable to their effects upon multiple pathways. Block of β1 receptors in the sinoatrial node reduces heart rate and block of myocardial receptors reduces contractility (reduced chronotropy and inotropy). They also reduce sympathetic nervous system activity and block of receptors in the juxtaglomerular apparatus reduces renin secretion. Some β-blockers block sodium channels and have membrane stabilizing activity and used as antiarrhythmic agent.

A. Timolol (Glucomol)

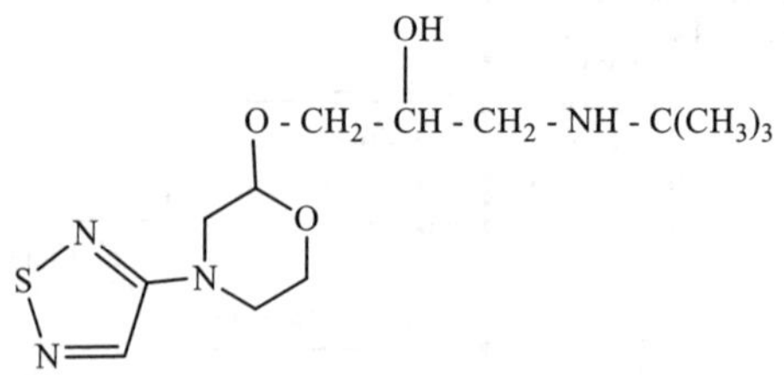

1- (t - Butylamino) - 3 - [(4 - morpholin - 4 - yl - 1, 2, 5 - thiadiazol - 3 - yl) oxy] propan - 2 - ol

It is a propanolamine derivative and possesses an asymmetric carbon atom in its structure and is provided as *levo* isomer.

Mechanism of action: It is a non-selective β-blocker. It competes with adrenergic neurotransmitters for binding to β_1-adrenergic receptors in the heart and the β_2-receptors in the vascular and bronchial smooth muscle. This inhibits the stimulatory effects of the sympathetic nervous system, reduce heart rate and contractility, peripheral vascular resistance and reduce the blood pressure.

Use: It is given in an eye drop solution to reduce intraocular pressure or pressure in the eyes. It is also used in tablet form as a drug to treat hypertension.

2.2 Adrenergic Neuron Blockers

Adrenergic neuron blockers act by interfering with adrenergic transmission. They may be classified into

- Drugs which prevent release of nor-adrenaline: eg. Guanethidine, Bretylium, Bethanidine
- Drugs that inhibit storage of nor-adrenaline: eg. Reserpine
- Drugs that interfere with synthesis of nor-adrenaline: eg. Metyrosine

A. Guanethidine monosulphate (Ismelin)

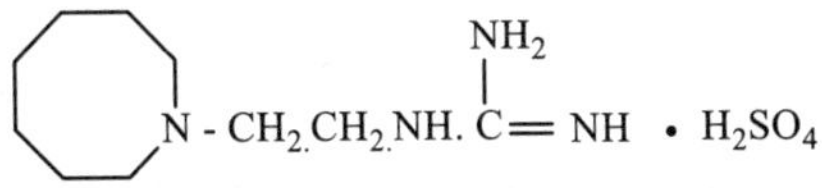

[2 - (Hexahydro - 1 - (2H) - azocinyl) ethyl] guanidine Sulphuric acid

It acts by interfering with adrenergic transmission

Mechanism of action: It is a postganglionic sympathetic nerve terminal blocker that prevents the release of nor-epinephrine from nerve terminals. It causes vasodilatation, increases venous capacitance, decreasing the heart rate and lower blood pressure.

Use: It is used as antihypertensive agent.

B. Reserpine (Diupres)

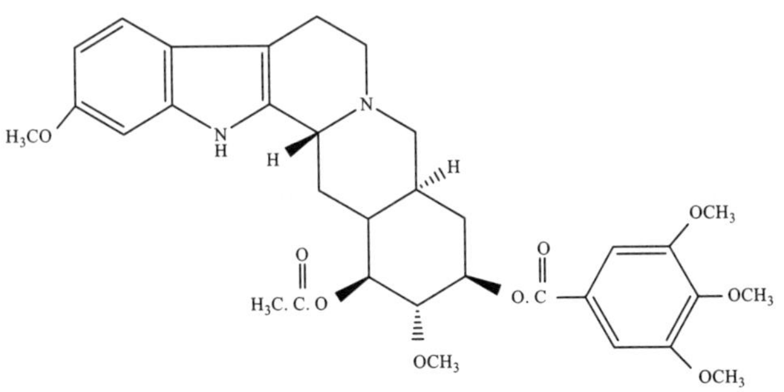

(3β, 16β, 17α, 18β, 20α,) - 11, 17 - Dimethoxy - 18 - [(3, 4, 5 - trimethoxy benzoyl) oxy] yohimban - 16 - carboxylic acid methyl ester

It is an indole alkaloid derived from the dried root of *Rauwolfia serpentina* (Indian snake root) and *Rauwolfia vomitoria.* It is a catecholamine-depleting sympatholytic agent.

Mechanism of action: It inhibits catecholamine pump on the storage vesicles in central and peripheral adrenergic neurons, thereby inhibiting the uptake of nor-epinephrine, dopamine and serotonin into presynaptic storage vesicles. This results in depletion of catecholamines and serotonin in central and peripheral nerve terminals. The antihypertensive action of Reserpine is due its ability to deplete catecholamine from peripheral sympathetic nerve endings.

Use: It is effective orally and parenterally for the treatment of hypertension.

2.3 Centrally Acting Agents

Methyldopa, Clonidine, Guanabenz and Guanfacine are drugs that exert their antihypertensive effect by stimulating α_2-adrenergic receptors in the brain stem. They interfere with sympathetic nervous system activity by stimulating brain-stem regulatory α_2-receptors. This reduces sympathetic outflow to the heart, thereby decreasing cardiac output by decreasing heart rate and contractility. Reduced sympathetic output to the vasculature decreases sympathetic vascular tone, which causes vasodilation and reduced systemic vascular resistance, which decreases arterial pressure.

A. Clonidine hydrochloride (Arkamin)

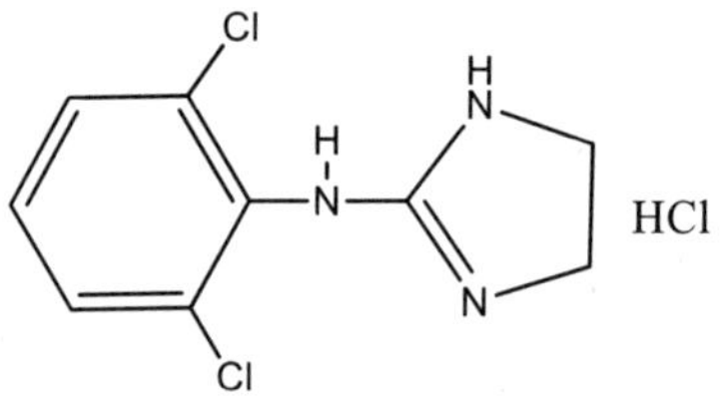

N - (2, 6 - Dichloro phenyl) - 4, 5 -dihydro -
1H - imidazol - 2 - amine hydrochloride

Clonidine is an example of phenyl-imino-imidazoline derivative that possesses selective α_2-adrenergic receptor.

Mechanism of action: It is a centrally-acting α-adrenergic agonist, with antihypertensive activity. It binds to central α_2-adrenergic receptors and thereby reducing the amount of nor-epinephrine release. This decreases sympathetic outflow to the heart, kidneys and peripheral vasculature. The reduction in sympathetic outflow leads to decreased peripheral vascular resistance, decreased blood pressure and decreased heart rate. In addition, clonidine binds to imidazoline receptor subtype-1, which may also contribute to a reduction in blood pressure.

Use: It is a selective α_2-adrenergic receptor. It is used as antihypertensive agent.

B. Methyldopate hydrochloride (Sembrina)

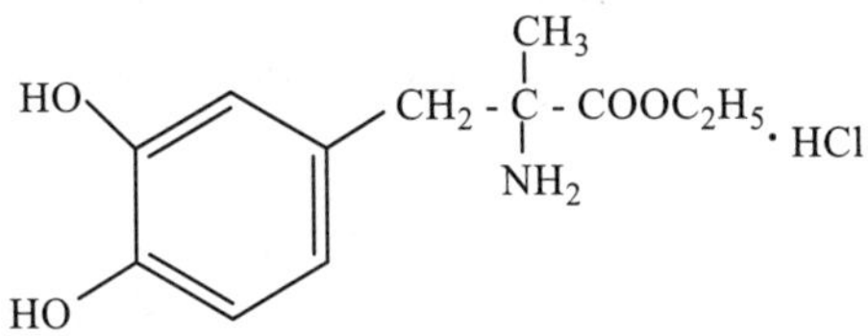

L - 3 - (3, 4 - dihydroxy phenyl) - 2 - methyl alanine ethyl ester hydrochloride

Synthesis

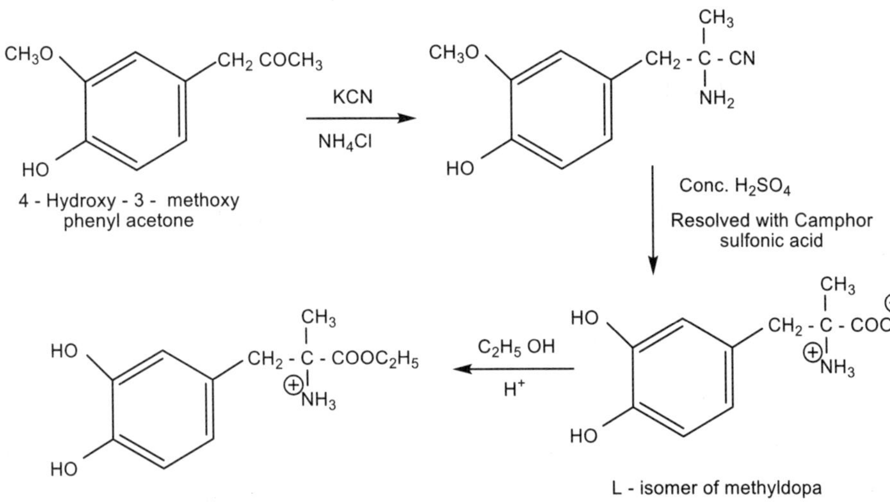

Methyldopa is an ethyl amine derivative that shows selectivity towards α_2- adrenergic receptor. It is a structural analogue of Dopa and function as a prodrug. After administration, it is converted into an active metabolite α-methylnor-epinephrine. It is an inhibitor of *aromatic-D-amino acid decarboxylase* (*Dopa decarboxylase*) and only L-isomer of Methyl dopa has the ability to inhibit *Dopa decarboxylase* and possess antihypertensive activity. D-Methyldopa is an inactive isomer of Methyldopa.

Mechanism of action: It act by the following mechanism

- Methyldopa is a prodrug which is metabolized to the active agent, α-methyl nor-epinephrine which acts in the brain, inhibiting adrenergic outflow from the brainstem. Inhibition of sympathetic outflow results in a decrease in blood pressure.

- It is an inhibitor of *aromatic-D-amino acid decarboxylase* which converts L-DOPA into dopamine. Dopamine is a precursor for nor-epinephrine and subsequently epinephrine. This inhibition results in reduced dopaminergic and adrenergic neurotransmission in the peripheral nervous system. This effect lower blood pressure.

Use: It is used in the treatment of hypertension and gestational hypertension (or pregnancy-induced hypertension)

C. Guanabenz acetate (Wytensin)

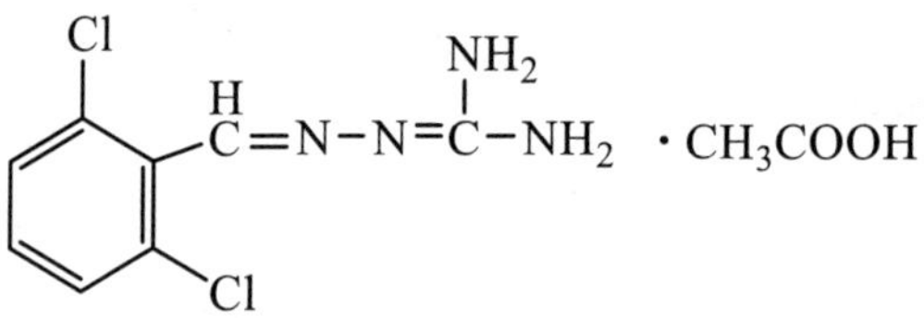

2 - {[(2, 6 - Dichlorophenyl) methylidene]amino}guanidine acetate

Mechanism of action: Antihypertensive effect of Guanabenz is due to central α-adrenergic stimulation, which results in a decreased sympathetic outflow to the heart, kidneys and peripheral vasculature in addition to a decreased systolic and diastolic blood pressure and a slight slowing of pulse rate.

Use: It is used as antihypertensive agents.

2.4 Vasodilators

Vasodilators are drugs that act directly on the arteriolar smooth muscle and decrease vascular resistance and arterial blood pressure. Since these drugs cause salt and water retention, it should be used in conjugation with diuretics and β-blockers.

Based on site of action vasodilators are classifies as

- **Arterial dilators:** They reduce arterial pressure by decreasing systemic vascular resistance. They are used to treat hypertension, heart failure and angina. eg. Nifedipine, Hydralazine, Minoxidil.
- **Venous dilators**: They reduce venous pressure, which reduces preload on the heart thereby decreasing cardiac output. This is useful in angina because it decreases the oxygen demand of the heart and thereby increases the oxygen supply/demand ratio. eg. Organic nitrates.
- **Mixed or Balanced dilators**: Most vasodilators act on both arteries and veins and therefore are termed mixed or balanced dilators. eg. Sodium nitroprusside, ACE inhibitors, Adrenergic blockers.

A. Hydralazine hydrochloride (Apresoline)

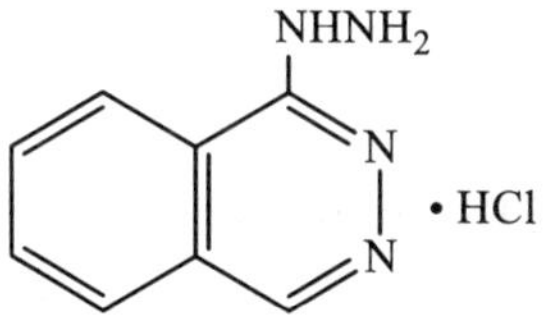

1- Hydrazino phthalazine

It is a hydrazine phthalazine class of drug

Mechanism of action: It is a direct-acting smooth muscle relaxant. By interfering with calcium transport, it relaxes arteriolar smooth muscle and decrease peripheral resistance, thereby lower blood pressure.

Use: It is used in the treatment of moderate to severe hypertension. A combination product with Isosorbide dinitrate is used as an adjunct therapy in the treatment of heart failure.

B. Minoxidil (Mintop, Gromane)

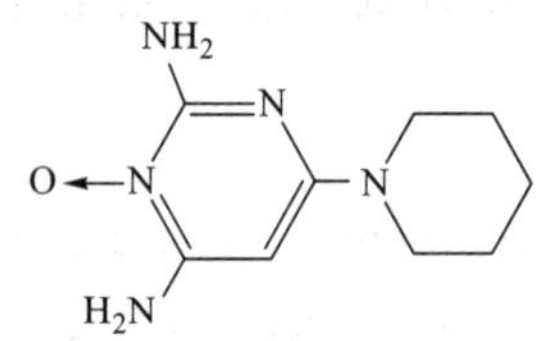

2, 4′- Diamino - 6 - piperidino pyrimidine - 3 - oxide

It is directly acting vasodilator. It is a prodrug and bio-transformed in liver by *sulfotransferase* into active Minoxidil sulfate.

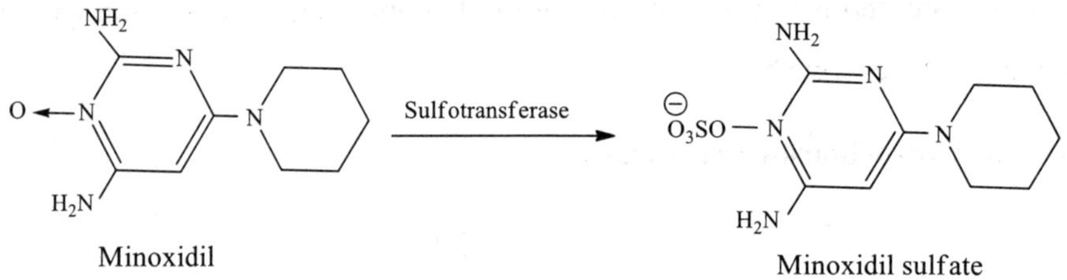

Mechanism of action: It is called as potassium channel opener. It activates ATP-sensitive potassium channel, which leads to decrease in intercellular Ca^{++} and reduces the excitability of smooth muscle and decrease peripheral resistance, thereby lower blood pressure. This vasodilation may also improve the viability of hair cells or hair follicles.

Use: It is used for severe hypertension that is difficult to control with another hypertensive agent. Topically it is used to treat androgenetic alopecia (Male pattern baldness).

C. Diazoxide (Eudemine)

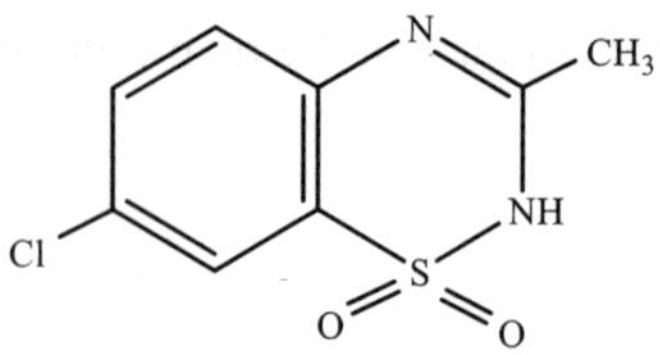

7 - Chloro - 3 - methyl - 2H - 1, 2, 4 - benzothiadiazine - 1, 1 - dioxide

It is a benzothiadiazine derivate and a potassium channel activator

Mechanism of action: It increases membrane permeability to potassium ions in vascular smooth muscle, thereby stabilizing the membrane action potential and preventing vascular smooth muscle contraction; this results in peripheral vasodilatation and decreases blood pressure. Diazoxide also inhibits the secretion of insulin by opening ATP-sensitive potassium channel of β-cells of the pancreas; thus, produce hypoglycemic effect.

Use: It is used as antihypertensive and hyperglycemic agent.

D. Sodium nitroprusside (Nitro press)

It is one of the most potent blood pressure lowering agents.

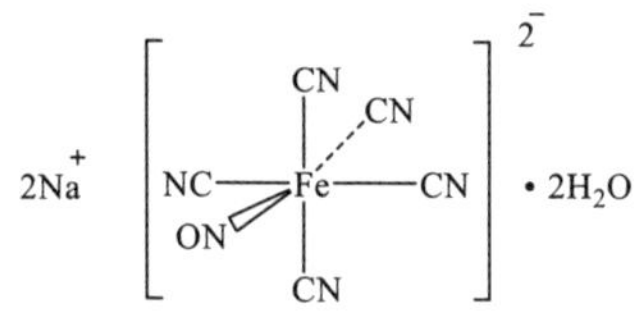

Sodium pentacyanonitrosyl ferrate (II)

It is a short-acting direct nitro vasodilator that is used intravenously for therapy of severe hypertension and heart failure. Sodium nitroprusside is water-soluble sodium salt usually a dihydrate, comprised of Fe^{2+} complexes with nitric oxide (NO) and five cyanide anions. It is sensitive to light, heat and moisture. Exposure to light causes deterioration that may be observed as a change in colour from brown to blue caused by reduction of the ferric ion to a ferrous ion.

Mechanism of action: It has the advantage of being both an arteriolar and venous vasodilator, thus reducing both preload and after load of the heart so that no increase in cardiac output occurs. In the body it functions as a prodrug, reacting with sulfhydryl groups on erythrocytes and release Nitric oxide (NO). The NO stimulates *guanyl cyclase* leads to increased production of intracellular cGMP, which stimulates calcium ion movement from the cytoplasm to the endoplasmic reticulum, reducing the level of available calcium ions that can bind to calmodulin. This ultimately results in vascular smooth muscle relaxation and vessel dilation. Other smooth muscle (eg. uterus, duodenum) is not affected.

Use: It is used for immediate reduction of blood pressure of patients in hypertensive crisis, reduces bleeding during surgery and for the treatment of acute congestive heart failure.

2.5 Targeting Renin-Angiotensin system

The renin-angiotensin system is a normal system that plays a role in the control of sodium excretion and body fluid volume. It interacts with sympathetic nervous system and aldosterone secretion in the regulation of blood pressure.

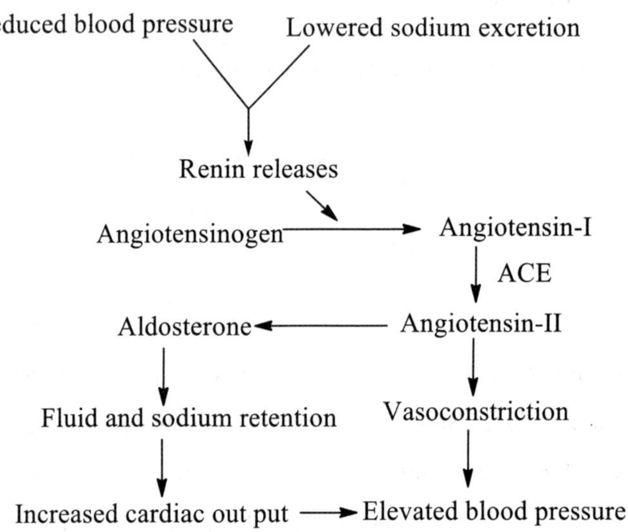

Fig. 5.1 Renin Angiotensin Pathway

Renin is *aspartate protease* endogenous enzyme that is secreted from the kidney due to internal stimuli. When there is a fall in blood pressure; reduced sodium level at the kidney and sympathetic nervous system stimuli secondary to a fall in blood pressure occurs. Renin converts Angiotensinogen to Angiotensin-I. (decapeptide). This in turn converted into Angiotensin-II (octapeptide) in the presence of ACE (angiotensin converting enzyme). Angiotensin-II is a potent vasodilator, as well as it stimulates adrenal gland to produce Aldosterone. Aldosterone increases blood volume and stimulate sodium reabsorption and potassium excretion. The net result is increase in blood pressure. Compounds which block ACE or bind to Angiotensin-II receptor are more effective antihypertensive agents. ACE inhibitors are also used in the treatment of congestive heart failure as first-line therapy. ACE also breaks down bradykinin (a vasodilator substance). Therefore, ACE inhibitors, by blocking the breakdown of bradykinin, increase bradykinin levels, which can contribute to the vasodilator action of ACE inhibitors.

2.5.1 ACE Inhibitors

ACE inhibitors produce vasodilation by inhibiting the formation of Angiotensin - II, the enzyme responsible for the conversion of Angiotensin - I to Angiotensin - II.
Based on the chemical structure it is classified as

(i) Sulfhydryl containing inhibitor: eg. Captopril.

(ii) Dicarboxylate containing inhibitors: eg. Enalapril, Lisinopril, Quinapril, Benazepril.

(iii) Phosphonate containing inhibitor: eg. Fosinopril.

2.5.1.1 Sulfhydryl Containing ACE Inhibitors

A. Captopril (Capoten)

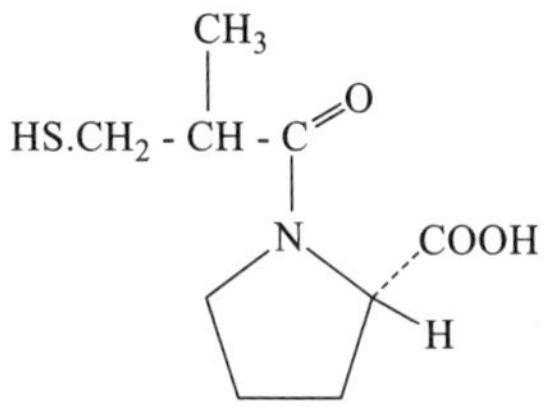

1- [(2S) - 3 - Mercapto - 2 - methyl - 1- oxo propionyl] proline

Mechanism of action: It is a potent, competitive inhibitor of Angiotensin-converting enzyme (ACE), the enzyme responsible for the conversion of Angiotensin-I to II. Angiotensin-II regulates blood pressure and is a key component of the renin-angiotensin-aldosterone system.

Use: It is used to treat hypertension, congestive heart failure, kidney problems caused by diseases.

2.5.1.2 Dicarboxylate containing ACE inhibitors

Table 5.1 Structures of ACE Inhibitors

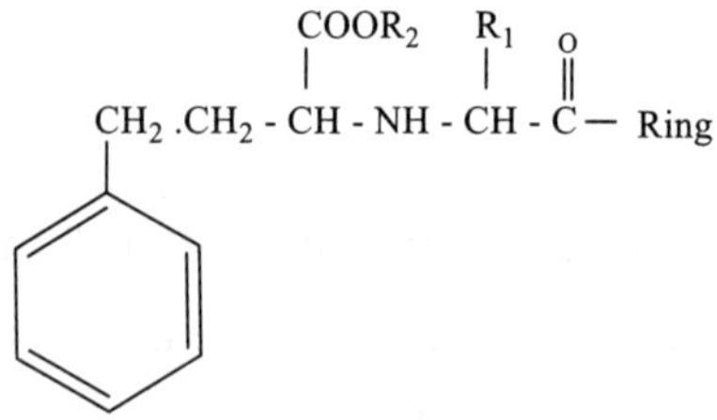

S. No.	Compound Name	R_1	R_2	Ring
1.	Enalapril	$-CH_3$	$-C_2H_5$	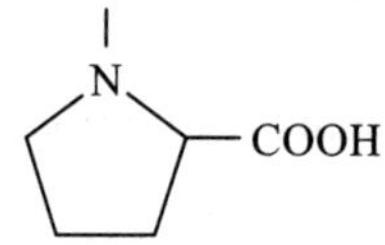
2.	Lisinopril	$-(CH_2)_4NH_2$	$-H$	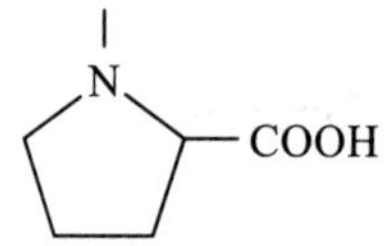
3.	Quinapril	$-CH_3$	$-C_2H_5$	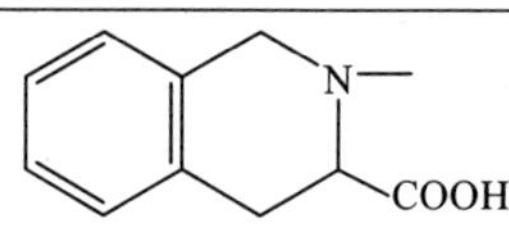

A. Enalapril (Enamate, Invoril)

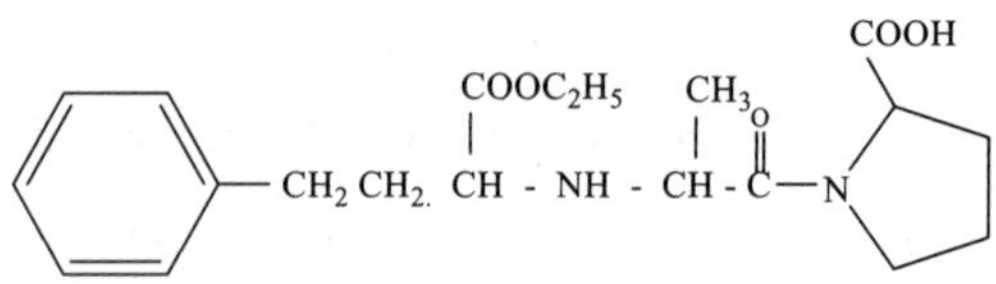

1- [N(S) - 1- Carboxy - 3 - phenyl propyl] - L - alanyl] - L - proline - 1' - ethylester

Enalapril is a prodrug of Enalaprilat. It is devoid of side effects of rash and loss of taste seen in Captopril.

Mechanism of action: It is hydrolyzed in the liver by *esterase* to active dicarboxylic acid enalaprilat. The active metabolite enalaprilat competitively binds to and inhibits ACE, thereby blocking the conversion of Angiotensin-I to Angiotensin-II. This prevents the potent vasoconstrictive actions of Angiotensin-II resulting in vasodilation.

Use: It is a long acting ACE inhibitor used in the treatment of reno vascular, essential and malignant hypertension and congestive heart failure.

B. Lisinopril (Linvas, Zestril)

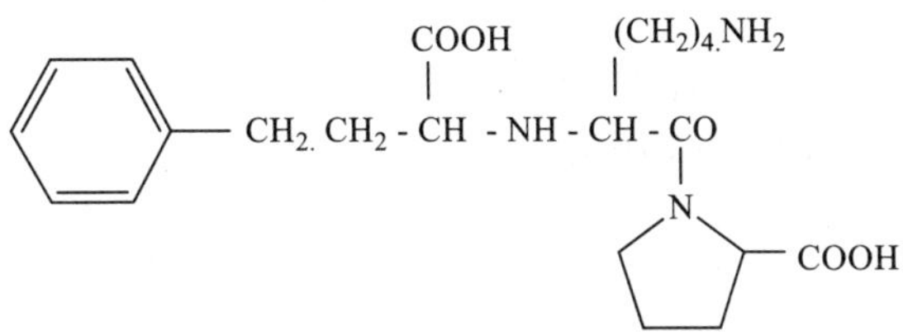

1- [N2 - (S) -1- carboxy - 3 - phenyl propyl] -
L - lysyl] - L - proline dihydrate

It is a lysine analogue of Enalaprilat

Mechanism of action: It competitively binds to and inhibits ACE, thereby blocking the conversion of Angiotensin-I to Angiotensin-II. This prevents the potent vasoconstrictive actions of Angiotensin-II resulting in vasodilatation.

Use: It is used in the treatment of renovascular essential and malignant hypertension and also for ventricular congestive heart failure.

C. Quinapril hydrochloride (Accupril)

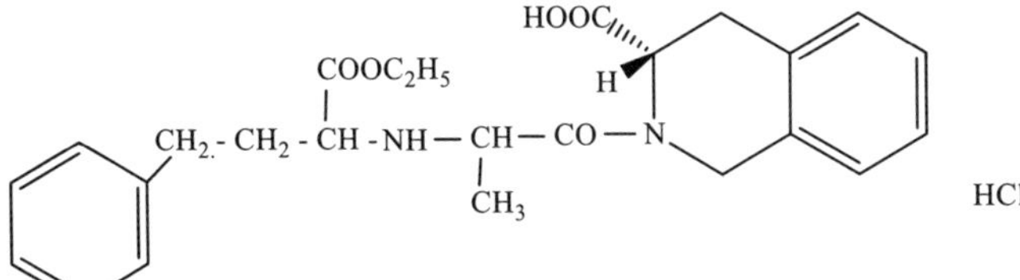

3S - [2(R(R) 3R] - 2 - {2 - [(1 - Ethoxy carbonyl) - 3 - phenyl propyl amino) - 1 - oxopopyl} - 1, 2, 3, 4 - tetrahydro - 3 - isoquinoline carboxylic acid hydrochloride

Quinapril hydrochloride is a tetrahydro isoquinoline analogue of Endopril.

Mechanism of action: It is a prodrug. Its active metabolite is Quinaprilat competitively binds to and inhibits ACE, thereby blocking the conversion of Angiotensin-I to Angiotensin-II. This prevents the potent vasoconstrictive actions of Angiotensin-II resulting in vasodilation.

Use: It is used as antihypertensive agent and also in the treatment of congestive heart failure.

D. Benazepril hydrochloride (Lotensin)

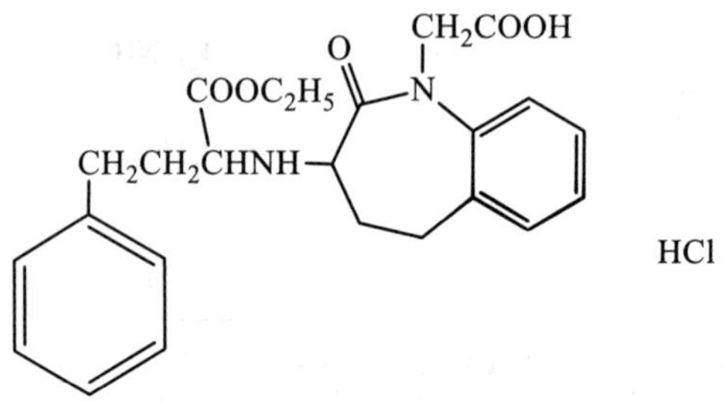

2 - [(3S) - 3 - [[(2S) -1- ethoxy -1- oxo - 4 - phenylbutan - 2 - yl]amino] - 2 - oxo - 4, 5 - dihydro - 3H - 1 - benzazepin - 1 - yl] acetic acid hydrochloride

Mechanism of action: As a prodrug, Benazepril is metabolized to its active form Benazeprilat competitively binds to and inhibits ACE, thereby blocking the conversion of Angiotensin-I to Angiotensin-II. This prevents the potent vasoconstrictive actions of Angiotensin-II resulting in vasodilation.

Use: It is used as antihypertensive agent and also in the treatment of congestive heart failure and chronic renal failure.

Chapter

6

ANTIARRHYTHMIC AGENTS

1. INTRODUCTION

Antiarrhythmic drugs are also known as cardiac dysrhythmia medications, are used to prevent and treat disorders of cardiac rhythm. Cardiac arrhythmias are abnormalities in the rate, regularity or site of origin of the cardiac impulse or a disturbance in conduction of the impulse such that the normal sequence of activation of atria and ventricles are altered. Arrhythmias appear to be predictive for sudden death.

2. CLASSIFICATION

Antiarrhythmic drugs are classified into four types according to their mechanism of action (Vaughan-Williams Classification)

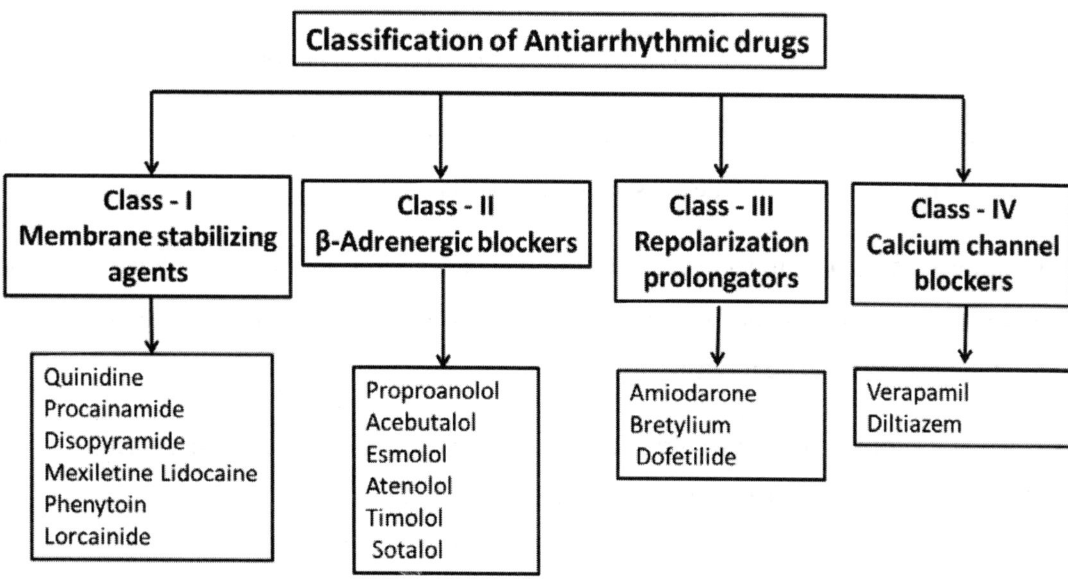

2.1 Membrane Stabilizing Agents

Class - I antiarrhythmic agents are drugs, that have membrane stabilizing properties (ie. they shift membrane to more negative potential).

2.1.1 Mechanism of action: Drugs in this class act in Na^+ channel and interfere with the process by which the depolarization charge is transferred across the membrane. These drug bind to Na^+ channel and block the rapid inwards sodium current, thereby slowing the rate of rise of action potential.

A. Quinidine sulphate (Qualaquin, Natcardin)

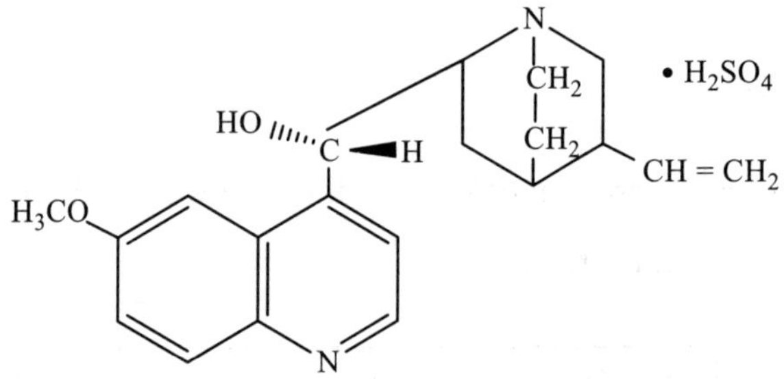

(8α, 9R) - 6' - Methoxy cinchonan - 9 - ol sulphate

It is an alkaloid isolated from cinchona bark. It is a *dextro* rotatory isomer of Quinine. The *levo* form Quinine is used as antimalarial agent.

Mechanism of action: It depresses excitability, conduction velocity and contractility of the myocardium and increases the effective refractory period, thus suppressing arrhythmic activity in the atria and ventricles.

Use: It is used to treat supraventricular and ventricular ectopic arrhythmias such as atrial ventricular tachycardia, atrial flutter and atrial fibrillation.

B. Procainamide hydrochloride (Pronestyl)

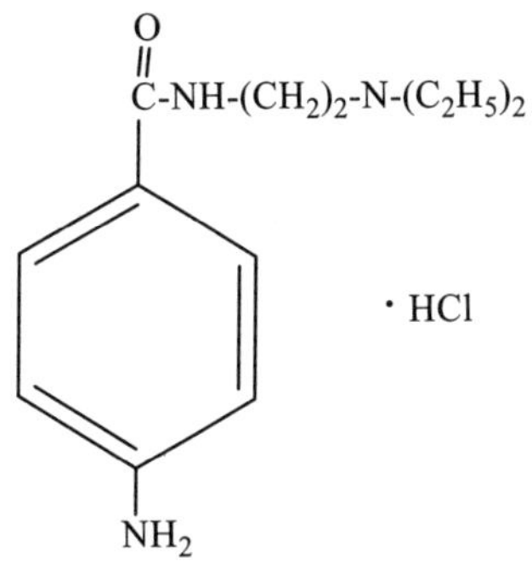

p - Amino - N- [2- (diethylamino) ethyl] benzamide hydrochloride

Mechanism of action: It is a sodium channel blocker. It stabilizes the neuronal membrane by inhibiting the ionic fluxes required for the initiation and conduction of impulses thereby effecting local anesthetic action.

Use: It is used as antiarrhythmic agent.

C. Disopyramide phosphate (Norpace)

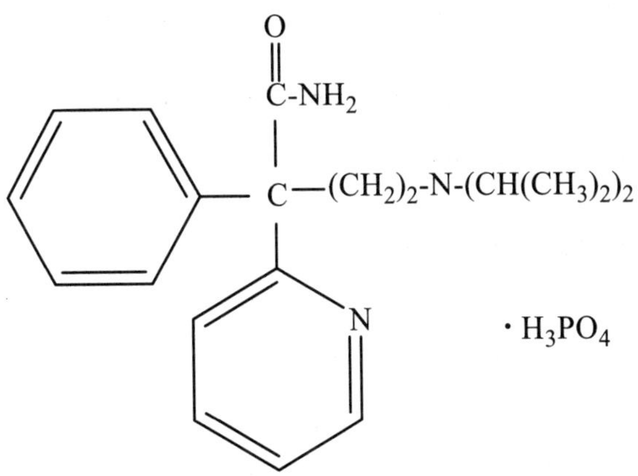

α - [(2) - Di-isopropylamino) ethyl] - α - phenyl - 2 - pyridine acetamide phosphate

It is available as phosphate salt. It is administered as a racemic mixture, but its antiarrhythmic activities reside on S-enantiomer.

Synthesis

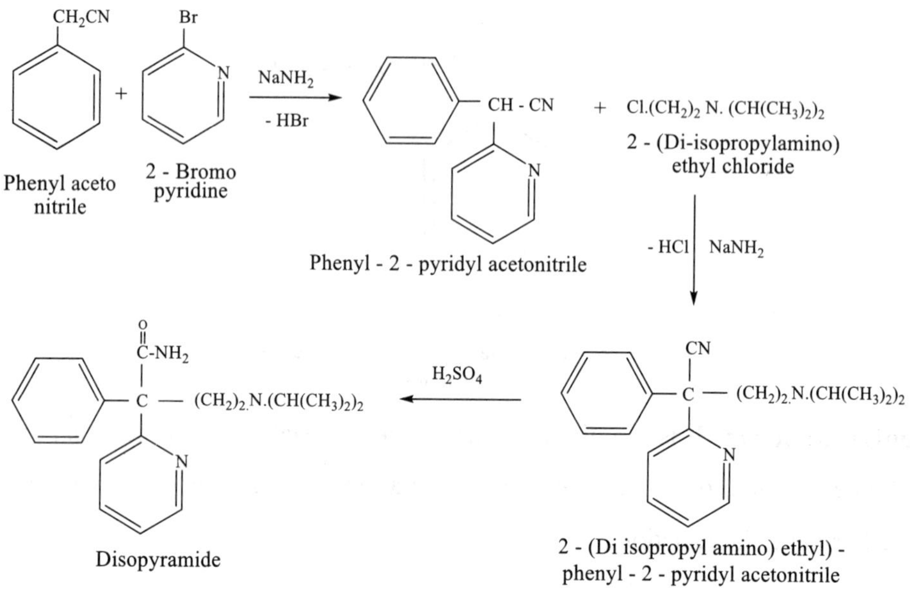

Mechanism of action: It is a class - I antiarrhythmic agent interferes directly with the depolarization of the cardiac membrane and thus serves as a membrane-stabilizing agent with a depressant action on the heart similar to that of Guanidine.

Use: It is an oral and intravenous class - I antiarrhythmic agent. It used in the treatment of refractory, life threatening ventricular tachyarrhythmias.

D. Lidocaine hydrochloride (Xylocaine)

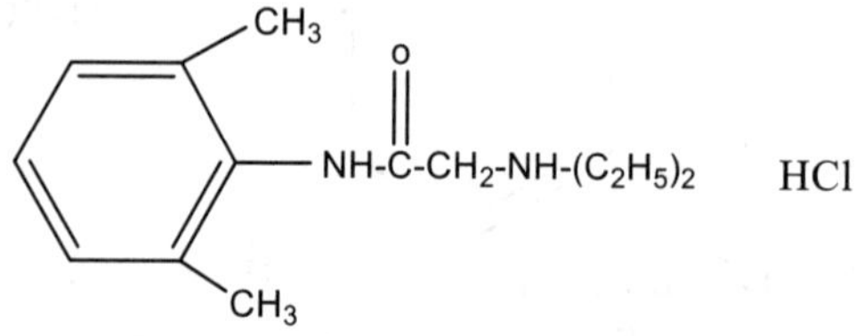

N,N - (Diethyl amino aceto) - 2, 6 - xylidine hydrochloride

It is also known as Lignocaine, is a local anesthetic of amide type. It is a synthetic aminoethyl amide with local anesthetic and antiarrhythmic properties.

Mechanism of action: It stabilizes the neuronal membrane by binding to and inhibiting voltage-gated sodium channels, thereby inhibiting the ionic fluxes required for the initiation and conduction of impulses and effecting local anesthesia. Blocking sodium channels in the conduction system, as well as the muscle cells of the heart, it acts as antiarrhythmic.

Use: It is a potent local anaesthetic agent reported to be twice as active as Procaine. It has local vasodilation action but usually used with vasoconstrictor adrenaline, to prolong the local anesthetic activity. It is used intravenously for the treatment of ventricular arrhythmias.

E. Phenytoin sodium (Eptoin, Epsolin)

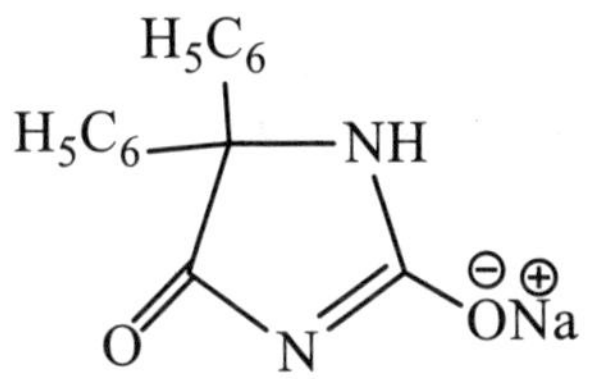

5, 5 - Diphenyl tetrahydro -1H - 2, 4 - imidazoledione sodium

It is a class - I antiarrhythmic agent. It is an antiepileptic drug and also a muscle relaxant.

Mechanism of action: It promotes sodium efflux from neurons located in the motor cortex, thereby stabilizing the neuron and inhibiting synaptic transmission. This leads to an inhibition of repetitive firing of action potentials and ultimately inhibits the spread of seizure activity.

Use: It is an antiepileptic drug useful against all types of seizures and also used as an anti-arrhythmic and muscle relaxant.

F. Mexiletine hydrochloride (Mexitil)

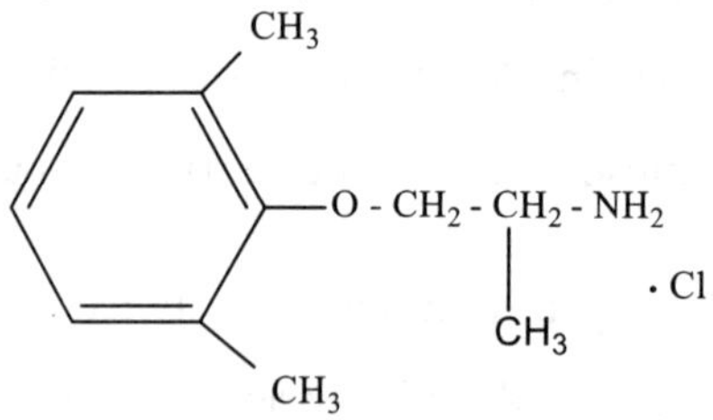

1- Methyl - 2 - (2, 6 - xylyloxy) ethylamine hydrochloride

Mechanism of action: It is a class - I antiarrhythmic agent.

Use: It is used for long term oral prophylaxis of ventricular tachycardia.

G. Tocainide hydrochloride (Tonocard, Tocolol)

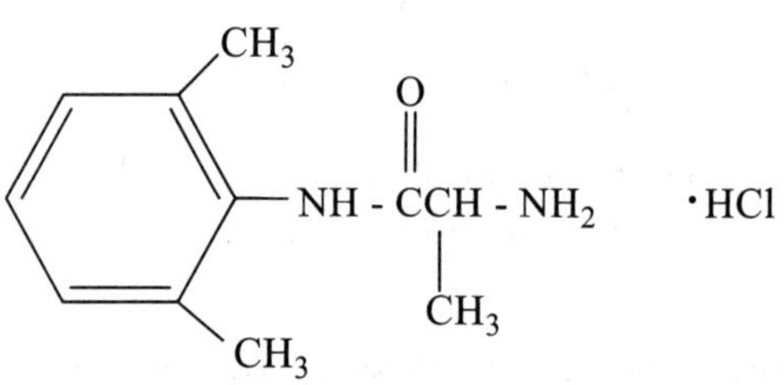

2 - Amino - 2', 6' - propionoxy xylidide hydrochloride

It is an analogue of Lidocaine

Mechanism of action: It is a class - 1B antiarrhythmic agent

Use: It is used to treat life threatening ventricular arrhythmias.

H. Lorcainide hydrochloride (Remivox)

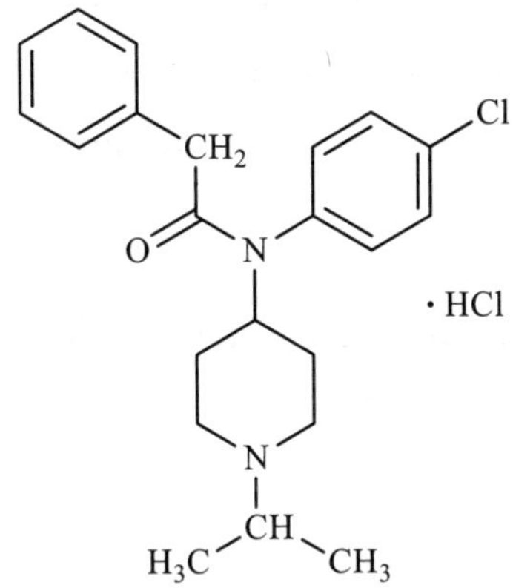

N - (4-Chlorophenyl) - 2- phenyl - N - (1-propan - 2-ylpiperidin - 4 - yl) acetamide hydrochloride

Mechanism of action: It is a Class-1C antiarrhythmic agent that is used to help restore normal heart rhythm and conduction in patients with premature ventricular contractions, ventricular tachycardiac and Wolff-Parkinson-White syndrome. It inhibits adenosine 5'-triphosphate (ATP) hydrolytic action of myocardial Na+K+*ATPase.*

Use: It is used for the treatment of ventricular arrhythmias, ventricular fibrillation and tachycardia

2.2 β - Adrenergic Blocking Agents

A. Sotalol (Sotagard, Solet)

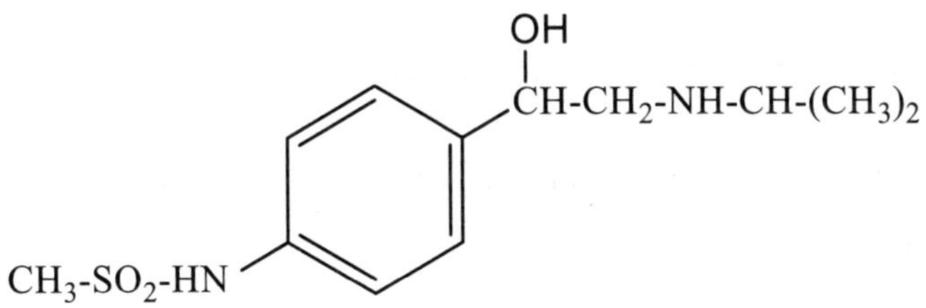

4'-(1- Hydroxy - 2 - (isopropyl amino) ethyl) methane sulfonanilide

It is a non-selective β-adrenergic blocker

Mechanism of action: It inhibits β_1-adrenoceptors in the myocardium as well as rapid potassium channels to slow repolarization and slow and shorten conduction of action potentials through the atria. The action of Sotalol on β-adrenergic receptors lengthens the sinus node cycle, conduction time through the atrioventricular node, refractory period and duration of action potentials.

Use: It is used for ventricular arrhythmias and maintaining normal sinus rhythm in atrial fibrillation or flutter.

2.3 Repolarization Prolongators

Class - III agents act by prolonging the action potential duration. Because potassium currents are normally responsible for repolarization of the cardiac action potentials. These agents are generally assumed to be potassium channel blockers. Member of this class prolong ventricular repolarization and increases the effective refractory period.

A. Amiodarone (Cordarone)

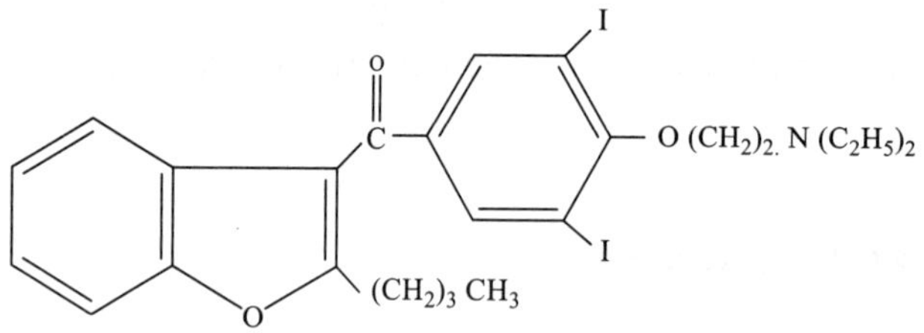

{2 - Butyl - 3 - benzofuranyl} - 4 - [2 - (diethyl amino) ethoxy] - 3, 5 - diiodophenyl ketone

It belongs to a class of drugs called Vaughan-Williams Class - III antiarrhythmic agents

Mechanism of action: The antiarrhythmic effect of Amiodarone is due to prolongation of myocardial cell-action potential (phase-3) duration and refractory period. It also acts as a noncompetitive α- and β-adrenergic inhibitor.

Use: It is used in the treatment of a wide range of cardiac tachyarrhythmia's, including both ventricular and supraventricular (atrial) arrhythmias.

Chapter 7

ANTIHYPERLIPIDEMIC AGENTS

1. INTRODUCTION

The pharmacological agent which reduces the concentration of plasma lipids are called hypocholesteremic agent or lipid-lowering agents. An increase in plasma lipids, particularly cholesterol is a common feature of atherosclerosis, a condition involving arterial damage which may lead to ischemic heart disease, myocardial infarction and cerebral vascular accidents. An increase in the plasma concentration of these substances is termed hyperlipidemia.

Lipids and cholesterol are transported through the blood stream as macromolecular complexes of lipid and protein known as lipoproteins. Lipoproteins are macromolecules consisting of lipid substances (cholesterol, triglycerides) non-covalently bound with protein and carbohydrates. These combinations solubilize the protein in the plasma. Lipoprotein consist of a central core of hydrophobic lipid (triglycerides or cholesteryl ester) encased in more hydrophilic coat of polar substances-phospholipid, free cholesterol and associated apoprotein. There are four main classes of lipoproteins differing in the relative proportion of the core lipids and in the type of apoprotein. They also differ in size and density and this property is measured by ultracentrifugation is the basis for this classification into:

- **Chylomicrons** transport triglycerides and cholesterol from the GIT to the tissues, where split by *lipase*, releasing free fatty acids further taken up in muscle and adipose tissue. Chylomicron are taken up in the liver
- **Very low density lipoproteins (VLDL)**, which transport cholesterol and newly synthesised triglycerides to the tissues, where triglycerides are removed as before leaving

- **Low density lipoproteins (LDL)** with a large component of cholesterol, some of which is taken up by the tissues and some by the liver, by endocytosis via specific LDL receptors
- **High density lipoproteins (HDL)** which absorb cholesterol derived from cell breakdown in tissues and transfer it to VLDL and LDL

Cholesterol is a lipid that is either absorbed from dietary sources or synthesized in the liver. It is an essential component of cell membranes allowing them to maintain permeability and fluidity. It is also required for the production of steroidal hormones and fat-soluble vitamins. Some forms of cholesterol can cause atherosclerosis (*LDL*) and therefore metabolizing cholesterol in an efficient manner is essential for health. The liver monitor cholesterol levels by altering the amount of production, absorption and bile secretion of cholesterol to maintain adequate level.

Plasma cholesterol concentrations are maintained by biosynthesis by the liver and extra hepatic tissues through the endogenous pathway and absorption of dietary and biliary cholesterol by the intestine through the exogenous pathway. Alteration of either pathway will affect the concentration of plasma cholesterol.

2. CLASSIFICATION

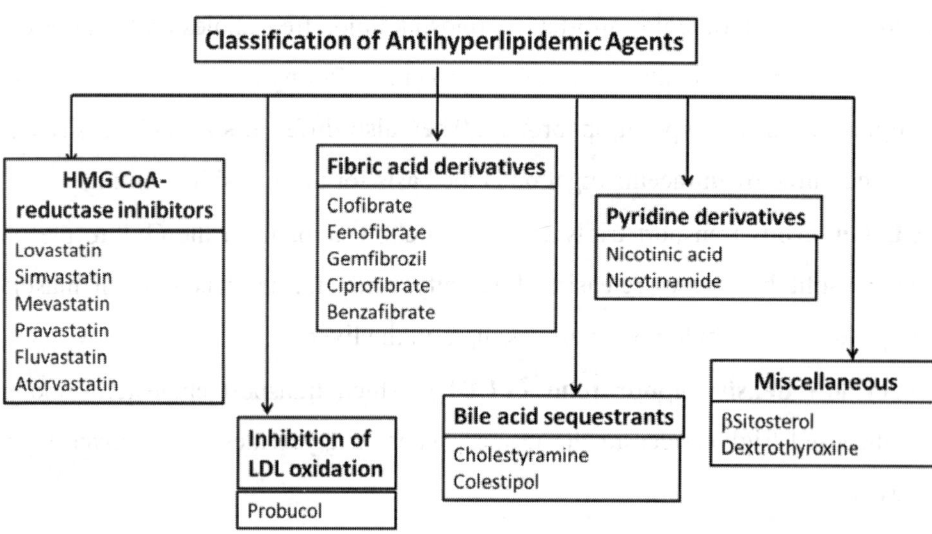

2.1 *HMG - CoA Reductase* Inhibitors

HMG-CoA is β-Hydro-β-methyl-glutaryl-CoA, is a substrate in the biosynthesis of cholesterol (Mevalonate pathway). *HMG-CoA reductase* is an enzyme that catalyzes the conversion of HMG-CoA to mevalonic acid. It is the rate-controlling enzyme of the mevalonate pathway, the metabolic pathway that produces cholesterol and other isoprenoids. Mevalonic acid is a required building block for cholesterol biosynthesis. *HMG-CoA reductase* inhibitors block the conversion of HMG-CoA to mevalonic acid in the synthetic pathway of cholesterol synthesis. These compounds are referred as statin.

Mechanism of Action

$$\text{Acetyl CoA} \xrightarrow[\text{NADPH}]{\textit{HMG - CoA reductase}} \text{Mevalonic acid} \longrightarrow \longrightarrow \text{Cholesterol}$$

Statins act by competitively inhibiting *HMG-CoA reductase*. Statins are similar to HMG-CoA at the molecular level. They bind to the enzyme, making it unavailable for the substrate. As a result, mevalonate is not formed; the next molecule in the cascade that eventually produces cholesterol. This ultimately reduces cholesterol by inhibiting cholesterol synthesis and increasing LDL uptake, overall lowering of plasma LDL level.

A. Lovastatin (Lova, Rovacor)

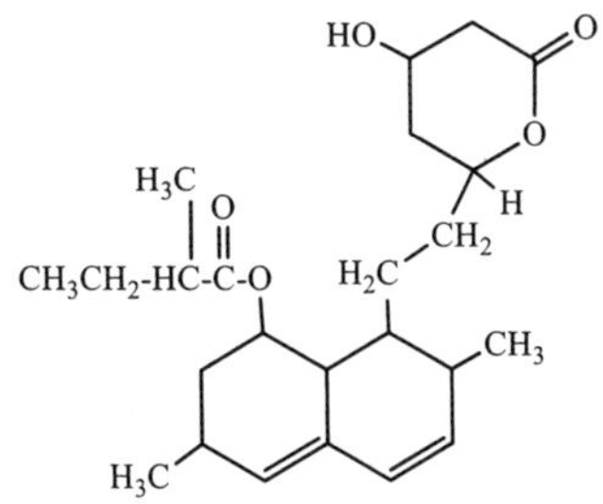

8 - {2 - [4 - Hydroxy - 6 - oxo oxan - 2 - yl]ethyl} - 3, 7 - dimethyl - 1, 2, 3, 7, 8, 8a - hexahydronaphthalen - 1 - yl - 2 - methylbutanoate

It is a naturally occurring drug found in food such as Oyster mushrooms and red yeast rice. It is obtained from the fermentation product of fungi *Aspergillus terreus* and

Monascus ruber. It is a prodrug and it must be hydrolyzed at lactone ring to open heptanoic acid for active metabolite.

Mechanism of action: It acts by competitively inhibiting *HMG-CoA reductase*.

Use: It is used in the treatment of dyslipidemia and the prevention of cardiovascular disease.

2.2 Fibric acid Derivatives

Fibric acid derivatives are regarded as broad-spectrum lipid lowering drugs. The main action is to decrease triglyceride levels, but they also tend to reduce low density lipoprotein (LDL) cholesterol levels and help to raise high density lipoprotein (HDL) cholesterol.

Mechanism of action: Fibrates appear to activate a protein called peroxisome proliferator-activated receptor alpha (PPAR-α). PPAR-α activates the enzyme lipoprotein *lipase* and ultimately results in decreased formation of very low-density lipoprotein (VLDL) cholesterol (which is converted into LDL cholesterol) and triglycerides and an increase in HDL cholesterol.

A. Clofibrate (Atromid-S)

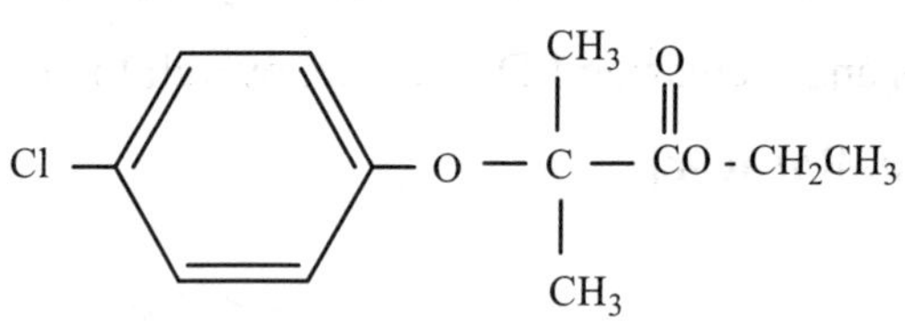

Ethyl - 2 - (4 - chloro phenoxy) - 2 - methyl propionate

It is an ethyl ester of clofibric acid and it is a prodrug

Use: It is an anticholesteremic agent used in the therapy of hypertriglyceridemia (Fredrickson types-IV and V hyperlipidemia).

2.3 Bile acid Sequestrants

The bile acid sequestrants are a group of resins used to bind certain components of bile in the gastrointestinal tract.

Mechanism of action: They are highly positive charged molecules that bind to the negatively charged bile acids in the intestine, inhibiting the lipid solubilizing activity and thus blocking cholesterol absorption. They also inhibit the reabsorption of bile acids and thus cause a contraction of the bile acid pool which leads to increased bile acid synthesis that competes with cholesterol synthesis in the liver. The body needs cholesterol to make bile, the liver uses up the cholesterol in the blood, which reduces the amount of LDL cholesterol circulating in the blood. These agents are used as hypolipidemic agents as an adjunct to the statins.

A. Cholestyramine (Questran)

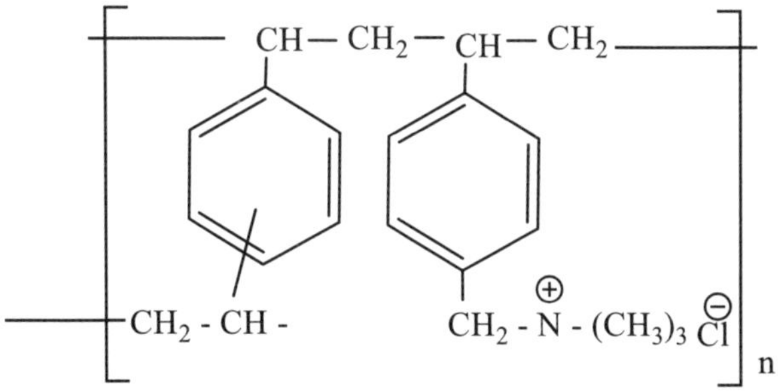

It is a styrene co-polymer with divinyl benzene with quaternary ammonium functional group. The resin is insoluble in water, remains unchanged in the intestinal tract, unaffected by digestive enzymes and is not absorbed. In small intestine, the Cholestyramine resin exchange chloride for bile acid, cationic ion exchange resin simply binds anionic bile acids. This form of insoluble complex result in increased loss of fecal bile acid and prevents its reabsorption into liver. The decrease in body content of bile acids is compensated by an increase in conversion of cholesterol to bile acids.

Use: It reduces cholesterol level without affecting triglycerides and effective in the treatment of type-III hyperlipoproteinemias.

B. Colestipol (Colestid)

Colestipol is a high-molecular weight, insoluble granular co-polymer of tetra-ethylene pentamine and epichlorohydrin. It functions as anion exchange resin sequestering agent in a similar manner.

Use: It reduces cholesterol levels without affecting cholesterol and it is also effective in the treatment of type-II hyperlipoproteinemias.

Chapter 8

COAGULANTS AND ANTICOAGULANTS

1. COAGULANTS

Coagulants or Hemostasis are drugs that promote coagulation and arrest bleeding. Coagulation or blood clotting is the process in which blood loses its fluidity and becomes a jelly like mass and it is a multistep process. The substances necessary for clotting are called clotting factors or procoagulants. Coagulation of blood is much more complicated and involves complex interactions between injured vessel wall, platelets and coagulation factors. A cascading series of proteolytic reaction is responsible for blood coagulation. Clotting may be initiated either by intrinsic or extrinsic pathway. Although both pathways are initiated by different mechanisms, the two converge on a common pathway that leads to clot formation. Coagulants may be used locally or systemically. Local homeostatic are called styptics. Some styptics used are adrenaline soaked in cotton, fibrin, thrombin powder and gelatin foam. Fresh plasma and whole blood are useful for most coagulation disorders as they contain all the clotting factors.

2. CLASSIFICATION

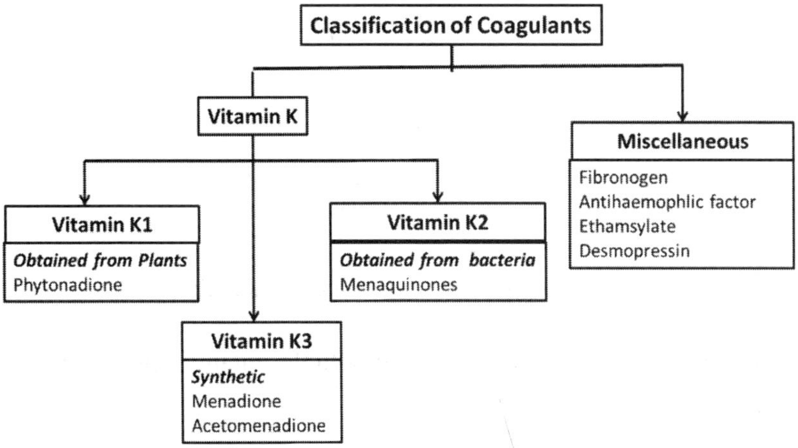

A. Menadione (Vitamin K_3)

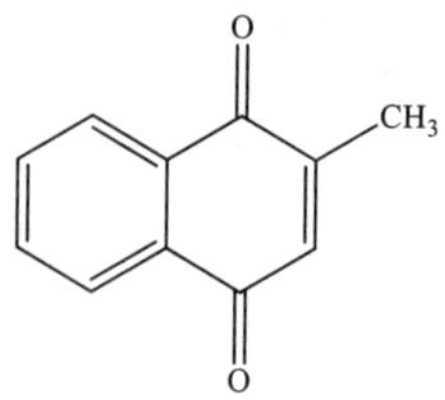

2 - Methyl - 1, 4 - naphthalenedione

Menadione is a synthetic fat-soluble vitamin precursor converted into active menaquinone after alkylation in the liver.

Mechanism of action: It acts as vitamin K analogues. Vitamin K acts as a co-factor in the synthesis of coagulation of proteins; prothrombin, factors VII, IX and X by liver. Vitamin K analogue is needed in the step of γ-carboxylation of these factors which are essential for coagulation cascade.

Use: It is used as a source of vitamin K. Because of cytotoxic side effects, it is no longer recommended as a dietary vitamin K supplement, although menadione is still commonly used in animal diets, partly in water-soluble form (eg. as menadione sodium bisulfite). It is used in the treatment of hypoprothrombinemia.

B. Acetomenaphthone (Vitamin K_4)

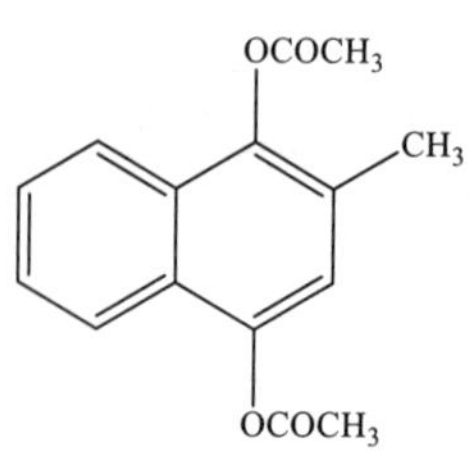

(4 - Acetyloxy - 3 - methylnaphthalene - 1 - yl) acetate

Acetomenaphthone is a diacetyl menadione

Mechanism of action: It is a synthetic, fat-soluble vitamin precursor converted into Menadione *in vivo*.

Use: It is used as a source of vitamin K.

3. ANTICOAGULANTS

3.1 Introduction

Anticoagulants commonly known as blood thinners, prevent the process of clotting, but do not break a clot that has formed already. Anticoagulants are usually administered to patient with acute myocardial infarction, long term therapy after acute myocardial infarction and prophylaxis and treatment of pulmonary and venous thrombosis.

3.2 Mechanism of Action

The coagulation of blood depends upon, cyclic inter-conversion of vitamin K and vitamin K-2, 3-epoxide. Vitamin K is a co-factor necessary for the post ribosomal synthesis of several clotting factors including II, VII, IX and X. The vitamin K sensitive step in this process involves the carboxylation of glutamate residues on the N-terminal portions of important precursor proteins. This carboxylation results in a new amino acid, γ-carboxy glutamate which through chelation of calcium ion causes the proteins to undergo a conformational change. This change in tertiary structure allows the four vitamin K dependent clotting factors to bind to phospholipid membranes during clotting cascade activation.

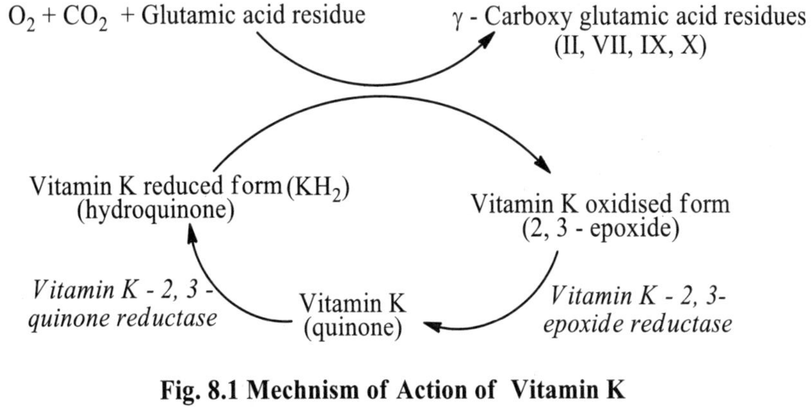

Fig. 8.1 Mechnism of Action of Vitamin K

The specific enzyme that carboxylates vitamin K dependent coagulation factors requires reduced vitamin K (**vitamin K hydroquinone**, KH_2), molecular oxygen and carbon dioxide as co-factors. In the process of this reaction, KH_2 is oxidized to vitamin K - 2, 3 - epoxide. The return of the epoxide to the active KH_2 form is the result of a two-step reduction. First, the epoxide is reduction to vitamin K quinone by *vitamin K - 2, 3- epoxide reductase* in the presence of NADH. This quinone intermediate is then further reduced back to KH_2 by *vitamin K quinone reductase.*

3.3 Classification

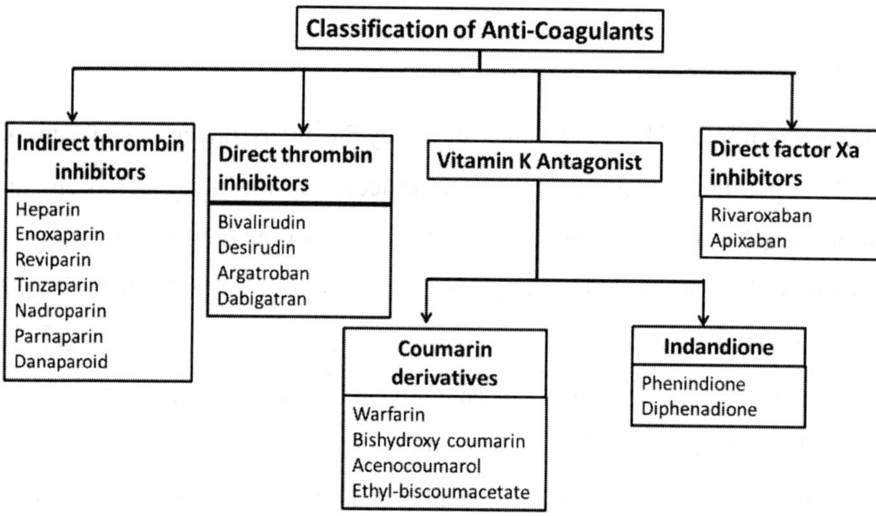

3.3.1 Coumarin Derivative

A. Warfarin (Waf)

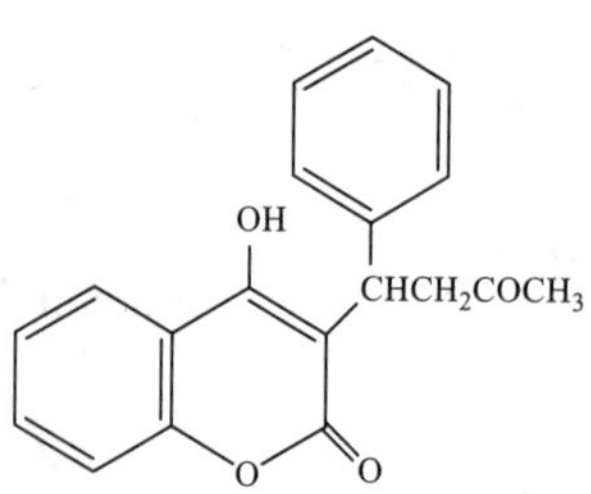

3 - (α - Acetonyl benzyl) - 4 - hydroxy coumarin

Warfarin forms a water-soluble derivative in alkali. Warfarin sodium (Coumadin) and Warfarin potassium they act by interfering with vitamin K metabolism. The (-) S isomer of Warfarin is five to eight times more active than (+) R enantiomer.

Synthesis

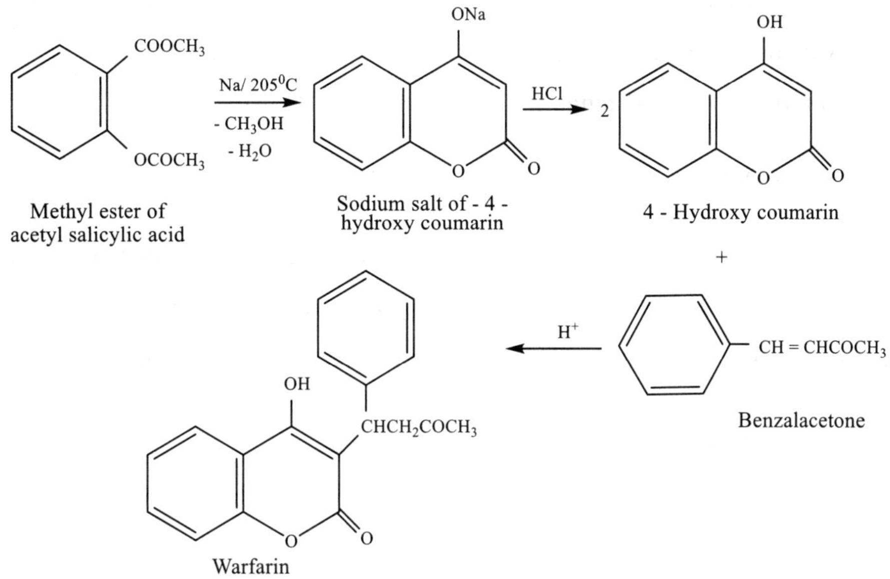

Mechanism of action: It is a vitamin K antagonist which inhibit the production of vitamin K by *vitamin-K-2, 3- epoxide reductase.* The reduced form of vitamin K, vitamin KH_2 is a cofactor used in the γ-carboxylation of coagulation factors VII, IX, X and thrombin. Carboxylation induces a conformational change allowing the factors to bind Ca^{2+} and to phospholipid surfaces. Uncarboxylated factors VII, IX, X and thrombin are biologically inactive and therefore serve to interrupt the coagulation cascade.

Use: It is a synthetic anticoagulant and also be used as rodenticides.

3.3.2 Indanedione Derivatives

A. Anisindione (Miradon)

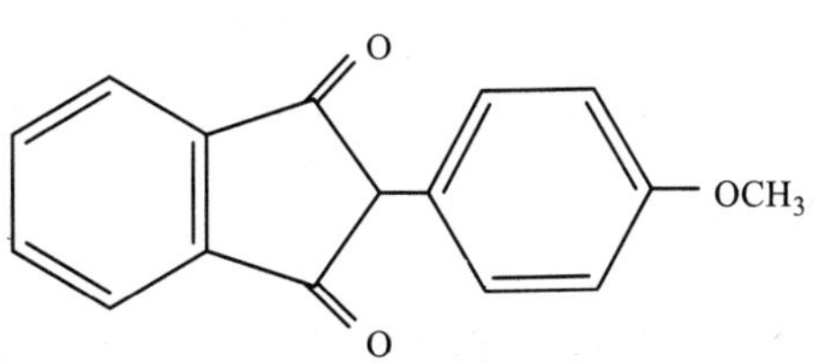

2 - (p - Methoxy phenyl) - 1, 3 - indandione

Mechanism of action: It acts as anticoagulant by inhibiting the vitamin K–mediated γ-carboxylation of precursor proteins, the formation of active procoagulation factors II, VII, IX and X as well as the anticoagulant proteins C and S is prevented.

Use: It is an orally active anticoagulant.

3.3.3 Antiplatelet Drug

It is also known as a platelet agglutination or aggregation inhibitor, is a member of a class of pharmaceuticals that decrease platelet aggregation and inhibit thrombus formation. They are effective in the arterial circulation, where anticoagulants have little effect.

A. Clopidogrel (Aptogrel, Clopid, Clopod)

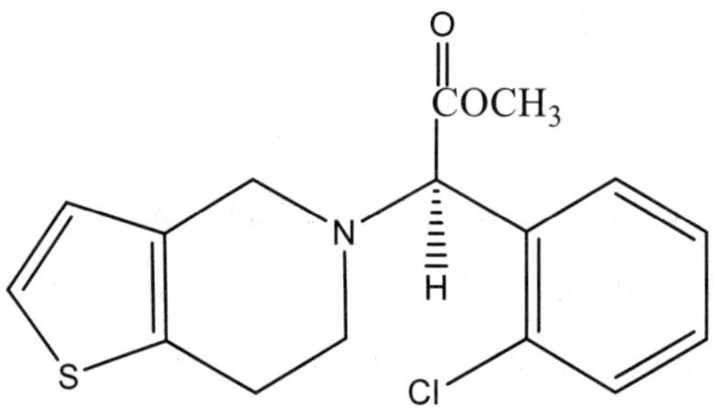

α - (2 - Chloro phenyl) - 6,7 - dihydro thieno [3, 2 - c] pyridine - 5 - acetic acide methyl ester

It is a prodrug with ester form. It is activated in the liver and due to opening of the thiophene ring the chemical structure of the active metabolite has 3 stereo centers, making a total of eight possible isomers. Only one of the eight structures with *Z*-configuration at the C_3-C_{16} double bond, the *S*-configuration at C_7 and *R*-configuration of the C_4 group is an active antiplatelet drug.

Mechanism of action: It is metabolized to its active form by *carboxylesterase-1*. The active form is a platelet inhibitor that irreversibly binds to ADP receptors on platelets and prevents activation of the glycoprotein complex and platelet aggregation.

Use: It is used in thrombosis prevention, in patient with atherosclerotic disease.

DRUGS FOR CONGESTIVE HEART FAILURE

Chapter 9

1. INTRODUCTION

Congestive heart failure (CHF) is a condition in which the heart is unable to pump enough blood to meet the metabolic needs of the body because of pathological changes in the myocardium. This condition can result from coronary heart disease, valve defects, lung disease, diabetes mellitus and hypertension.

Cardiac failure occurs when the heart is unable to pump blood effectively at a rate that meets the needs of the body. The heart muscle can perform only weakly, particularly on ventricular contraction. This reduced pumping capacity results in a reduced heart output. However, as new blood continues to enter the heart, the volume of blood in the heart increases. As the heart is unable to pump this blood out, it becomes congested, hence 'congestive heart failure'. This causes decrease in systemic blood flow, in turn reduces blood flow to the kidneys which stimulate the release of renin and aldosterone result in work load increase on the heart (Fig 9.1).

CHF is classified as

- Left heart failure (LHF) - leads to pulmonary edema and resulting dyspnea,
- Right heart failure (RHF) - induces systemic venous congestion that causes symptoms such as jugular venous swelling and hepatomegaly.
- Biventricular CHF - manifests with RHF and LHF, as well as general symptoms such as tachycardia, fatigue and nocturia.
- Acute decompensated heart failure (ADHF) - caused by an acute cardiac condition such as myocardial infarction.

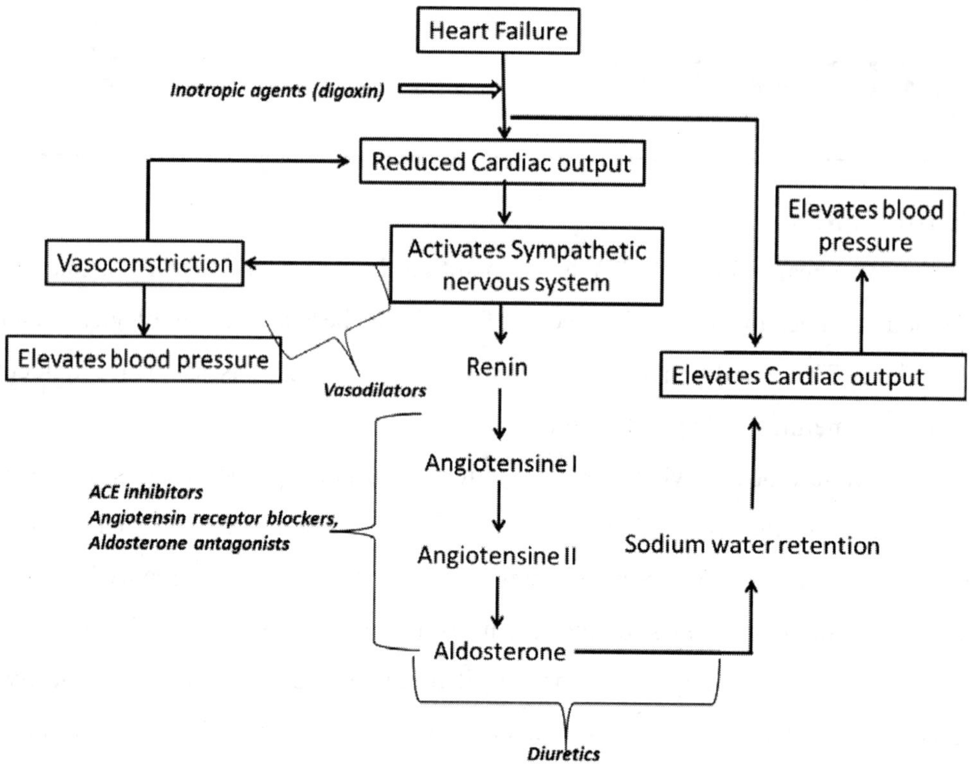

Fig 9.1 Pathophysiology of Congestive heart failure

2. CLASSIFICATION

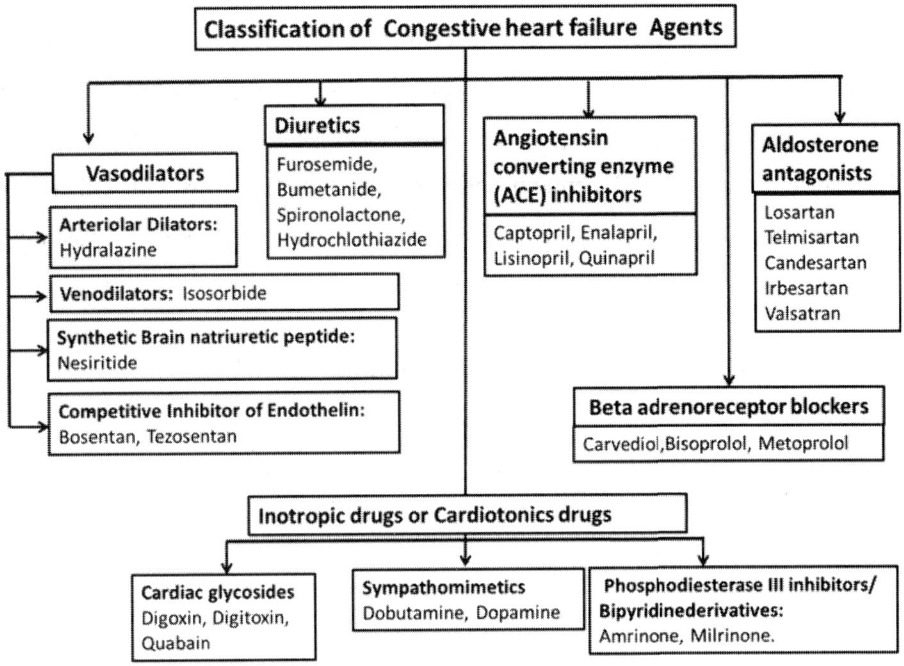

2.1 Inotropic Drugs

2.1.1 Cardiac Glycosides

Cardiac glycosides are glycosides containing a steroidal aglycone and have highly specific and powerful action on cardiac muscle. They are also called cardio-active glycosides and cardiotonic glycosides. The principle sources of cardiac glycosides are plant sources of cardiac glycosides are *Digitalis purpurea,* Digitalis lanata, *Strophanthus gratus* and *Strophanthus kombe.* Among all, *D. purpurea* and *D. lanata* are main sources of cardiac glycosides. Digitoxin and Digoxin are the glycosides which are frequently employed as medicine.

2.1.1.1 Chemistry of Cardiac Glycosides

All glycosides consist of an aglycone (genin) part to which are attached one or more sugar moieties (glycone). The cardiac activity resides in the aglycone portion, but the sugar moiety provides favorable solubility and distribution characteristics. On hydrolysis (acid or alkali or enzymatic) yield the corresponding steroidal aglycone and glycone (sugar). Structurally, cardiac glycosides consist of cyclopentano perhydro phenanthrene ring with either a 5- or 6-membered lactone ring attached at the 17th position and sugars attached at the 3rd position.

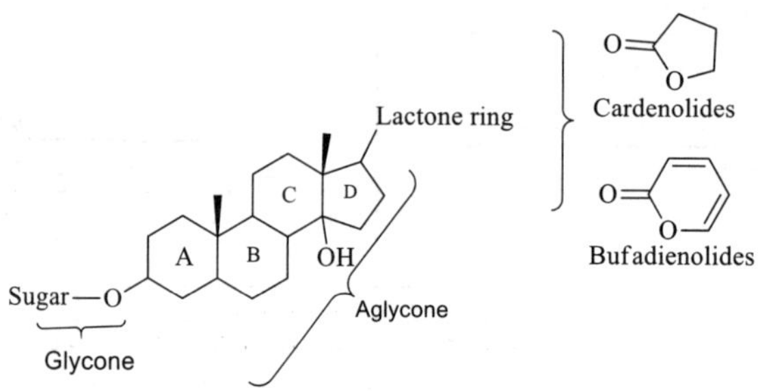

General structure of Cardiac Glycosides

i) **Aglycone**

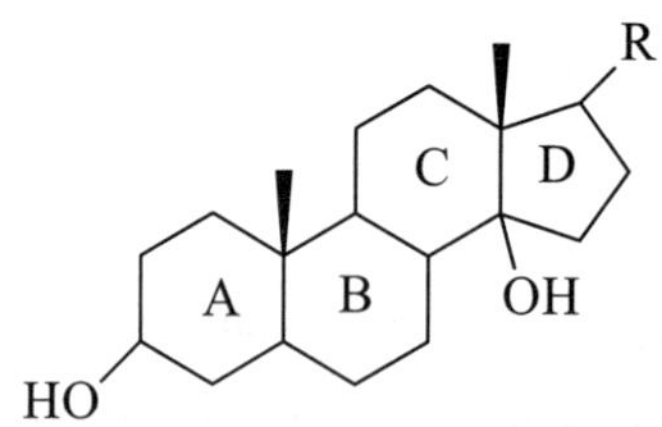

- Cardio tonic activity of the glycoside resides on aglycone part.
- Aglycone portion consist of cyclopentano perhydrophenanthrene (steroid) nucleus with a unique set of fused rings.

- Ring A/B and C/D are *cis* fused, whereas ring B/C have a *trans* configuration (the adrenocortical steroids typically possess an A/B, B/C and C/D all having *trans* conformation, while the bile salts characteristically have an A/B cis and B/C *trans* orientation).
- The steroidal nucleus carries two angular methyl groups at C_{10} and C_{13}.
- The hydroxyl group at 3rd position is the site of attachment for the sugar portion.
- The C_{14} hydroxyl group is normally unsubstituted; however additional hydroxyl group may be found at C_{12} and C_{16}. The presence or absence of which distinguishes the important genus like Digitoxigenin, Digoxigenin and Gitoxigenin.
- The size of the unsaturated lactone ring at C_{17} position varies with the source of glycoside. According to the type of unsaturated lactone ring attached to the C_{17} position of the cardiac glycoside, the cardiac glycoside canbe classified into two types:
  - Cardenolides
  - Bufadienolides

Cardenolides are 5-membered, α, β-unsaturated lactone (butyro lactone) ring, mostly occur in plants. Bufadienolides are 6-membered (α-pyrone) lactone ring with 2 conjugated double bonds and of animal origin. Pharmacologically, both have similar properties. The type of glycoside and the name of the structural components of these glycosides are tabulated in Table 9.1. The cardiac glycosides from animal source (generally bufadienolides) have less medicinal importance because of their high toxicity. Pharmaceutical preparations of whole plants and partially hydrolyzed glycosides of *Digitalis lanata* and *Digitalis purpurea* have been widely used clinically. Some aglycones of cardiac glycosides are used for congestive heart failure and commercially available are Digoxigenin, Gitoxigenin, Strophanthidin and Ouabagenin.

Table 9.1 Structures of Aglycone

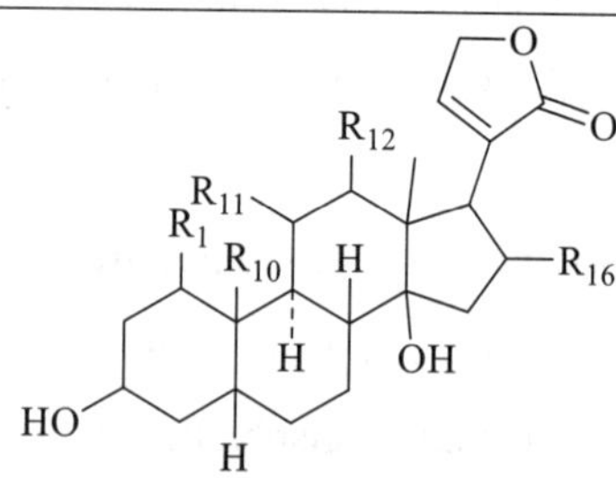

Aglycone	R_1	R_{10}	R_{11}	R_{12}	R_{16}
Digitoxigenin	-H	$-CH_3$	-H	-H	-H
Digoxigenin	-H	$-CH_3$	-H	-OH	-H
Gitoxigenin	-H	$-CH_3$	-H	-H	-OH
Ouabagenin	-OH	$-CH_2OH$	-OH	-H	-H
Strophanthidin	-H	-CHO	-H	-H	-H

ii) Glycone

The sugars found in the cardiac glycosides are D-Glucose, D-Digitoxose, L-Rhamnose, D-Cymarose, D-Digitalose, L-Thevetose, L-Oleandrose and D-Sarmentose. The number and the identity of sugar moiety vary from one glycoside to another. The sugar usually exists in β-configuration. The sugar (mono or polysaccharide) portion conjugates with the C-3 hydroxy group of the aglycone portion with β-1, 4-glucosidic linkages. Common monosaccharides found in cardiac glycosides are glucose, rhamnose and 6-deoxy monosaccharide. Although the sugar moiety does not have a cardiotonic effect, it can affect the pharmacokinetic properties of the cardiac glycosides.

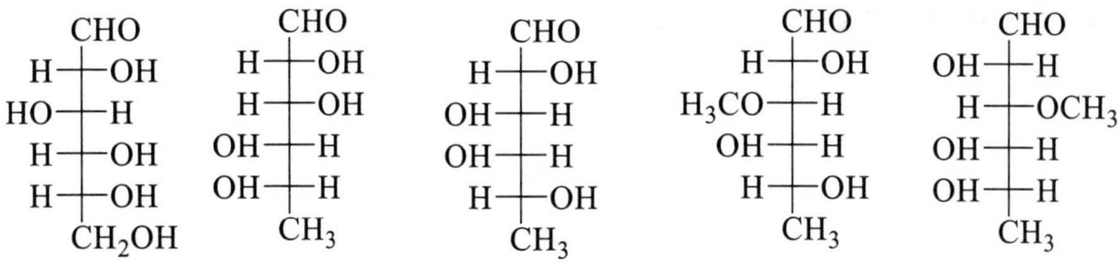

D-Glucose D-Rhamnose D-Glucomethylose D-Digitalose D-Thevetose

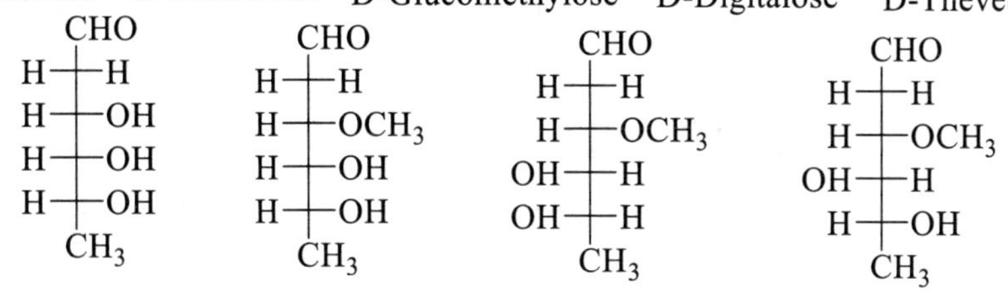

D-Digitoxose D-Cymarose D-Oleandrose D-Sarmentose

The glycoside present in *Digitalis lanata* and *Digitalis purpurea* are

Glycosides	Aglycone	Glycone
Digoxin	Digoxigenin	3 molecules of digitoxose
Digitoxin	Digitoxigenin	3 molecules of digitoxose

Mechanism of action: Cardiac glycosides exert a positive inotropic effect on the heart in cardiac failure.They increase the output force of the heart and increase its rate of contractions by inhibiting sodium-potassium *ATPase* pump, thereby increasing intracellular calcium and enhancing cardiac contractility.

Use: Cardiac glycosides are used to slow down the heart rate in atrial arrhythmias, particularly atrial fibrillation. They are also given in congestive heart failure.

A. Digoxin (Digitran, Sangoxin)

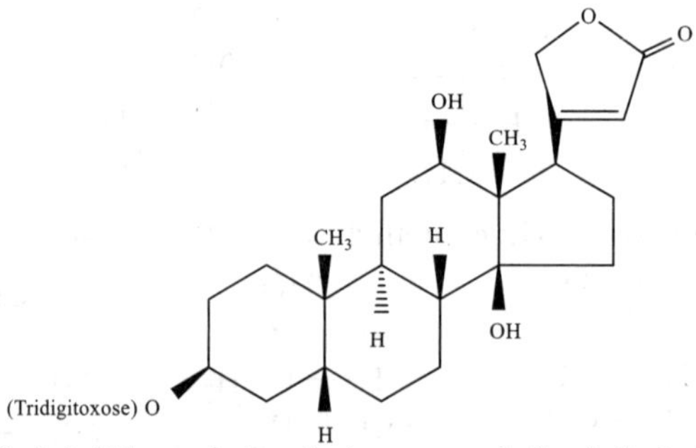

3β - [(O - 2, 6 - Dideoxy - β - D - *ribo* -hexopyronosyl - (1⟶4) - O - 2, 6 - dideoxy - β - D - *ribo* hexopyronosyl - (1⟶4) - O - 2, 6 - Dideoxy - β - D - *ribo* hexopyronosyloxy - 12β, 14 - dihydroxy - 5β, 14β - card - 20(22) - enolide

Digoxin is a cardiac (or digitalis) glycoside extracted from the leaves of foxglove plant, *Digitalis lanata* and *Digitalis orientalis.* It differs from Digitoxin in that it has an additional hydroxyl group at C_{16} of the steroid skeleton. It has positive inotropic and negative chronotropic activity.

Use: It is used in the treatment of congestive heart failure with atrial fibrillation.

B. Digitoxin (Chavuin)

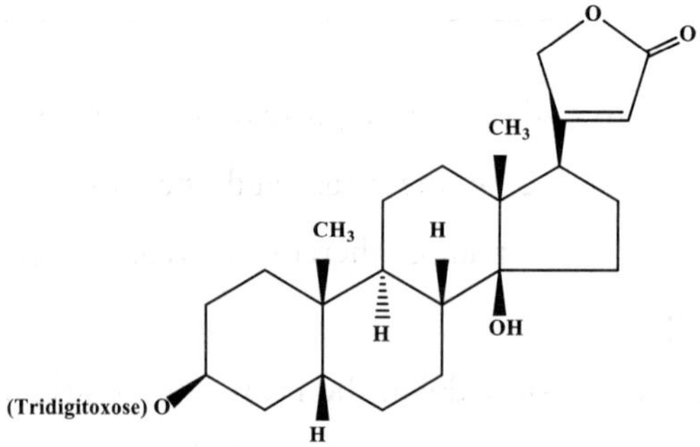

3β - [(O - 2,6- Dideoxy - β - D - ribohexopyranosyl (1⟶ 4) - O - 2,6- dideoxy - β - D - ribohexopyranosyl (1⟶ 4) - O - 2,6- dideoxy - β - D - ribohexopyranosyloxy) - 14 - hydroxy - 5β, 14β - card - 20 (22) - enolide

Digitoxin is 3β, 14β - dihydroxy-5β-card-20(22)-enolide-3-tridigitoxide, is a glycoside isolated from leaves of various types of foxgloves. It is sometimes used in place of Digoxin. It has a longer half-life than Digoxin.

Use: It is used in the treatment of congestive heart failure with atrial fibrillation.

2.2 Vasodilators

2.2.1 Synthetic Brain Natriuretic Peptide

A. Nesiritide (Natrecor)

It is a 32 amino acid containing recombinant human B-type natriuretic peptide (hBNP) and is manufactured from *Escherichia coli* using recombinant DNA technology.

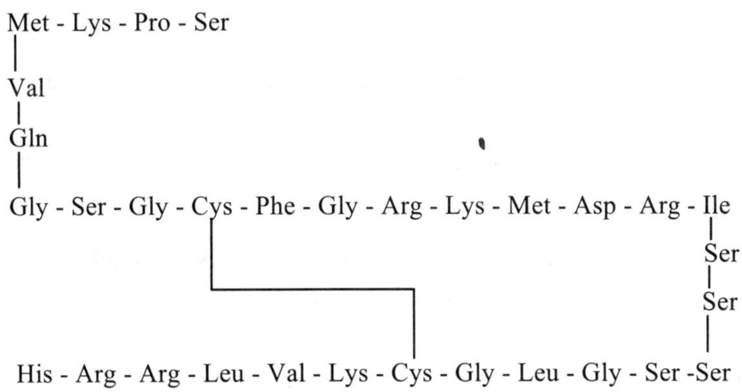

Mechanism of action: It activates *guanylyl cyclase* to form the potent vasodilator cGMP. Administration of the drug leads to balanced vasodilation in the arteries and veins, diuretic effects (via enhanced Na^+ excretion), suppression of the RAA system and suppression of the sympathetic nervous system.

Use: It is used to treat acute congestive heart failure.

2.2.2 Competitive Inhibitor of Endothelin

A. Bosentan (Tracleer)

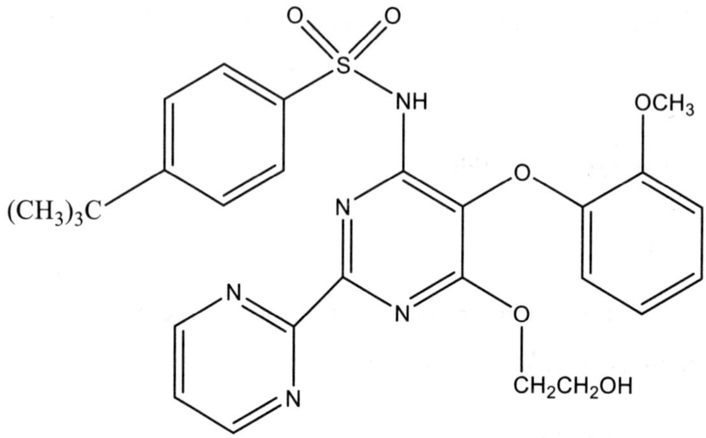

4 - (*Tert* - butyl) - *N* - (6 - (2 - hydroxy ethoxy) - 5 - (2 -methoxy phenoxy) - [2, 2' - bipyrimidin] - 4 -yl) benzene sulfonamide

Mechanism of action: It belongs to a class of drugs known as endothelin receptor antagonists (ERAs). Pulmonary arterial hypertension (PAH) has elevated levels of endothelin, a potent blood vessel constrictor, in plasma and lung tissue. Bosentan blocks the binding of endothelin to its receptors, thereby negating endothelin's deleterious effects.

Use: It is used to treat moderate pulmonary arterial hypertension.

B. Tezosentan (Veletri)

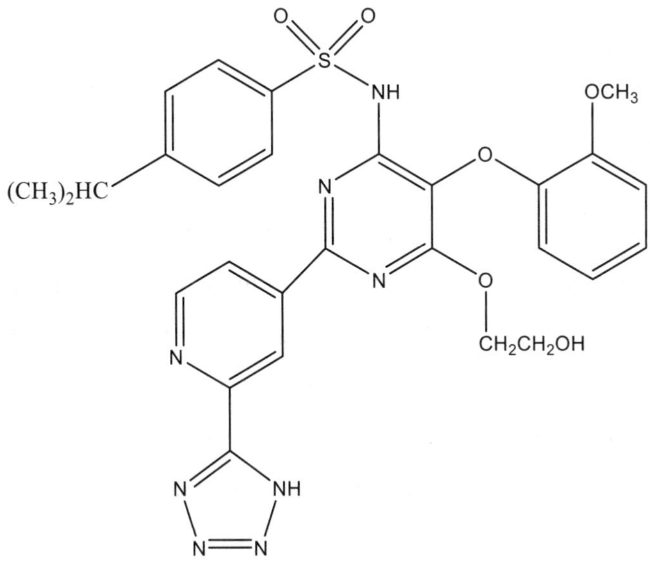

N - [6 - (2 - Hydroxy ethoxy) - 5 - (2 - methoxy phenoxy) - 2 - [2 - (2H - 1, 2, 3, 4 -tetrazol - 5 - yl) pyridin - 4 - yl] pyrimidin - 4 - yl] - 5 - (propan - 2 - yl) pyridin - 2 -sulfonamide

It belongs to the class of organic compounds known as pyridinyl-pyrimidines. It contains a pyridinyl-pyrimidine skeleton, which consists of a pyridine linked (not fused) to a pyrimidine by a bond.

Mechanism of action: It is a non-selective endothelin receptor antagonist. It acts by association with G-proteins that activate a phosphatidyl-inositol-calcium second messenger system.

Use: It is used for the treatment of congestive heart failure, liver disease and heart disease.

Chapter

10

STEROIDAL HORMONES

1. INTRODUCTION

Steroids are a class of substances, which are widely distributed in animals and plants. In humans, all steroid hormones are derived from cholesterol. They are produced by certain endocrine organs and released into the bloodstream to reach target cells. The steroidal hormones regulate many physiologic processes, including carbohydrate regulation (glucocorticoids), mineral balance (mineralocorticoids) and the development and function of the reproductive system (gonadal steroids). Steroids also play roles in inflammatory responses, stress responses, bone metabolism, cardiovascular fitness, behavior, cognition and mood. Steroids are lipid soluble in nature and thus are freely permeable to membranes so are not stored in cells.

Steroidal hormones are classified into two types

I. Sex hormones

II. Adrenal cortical hormones

Steroidal hormones are produced and secreted at two major places in the human body: the adrenal glands and the gonads (the testes in males and the ovaries in females). Adrenal glands are present at the top of each kidney. An outer layer of the gland, the adrenal cortex, produces a number of potent steroidal hormones. The adrenal cortex steroids are often called adrenal corticoids or simply corticoids.

1.1 Structure and Stereochemistry

All steroids possess cyclopentano perhydrophenanthrene (Sterane) nucleus as common basis structure. It consists of three fused rings known as phenanthrene (rings A, B, and C) and the cyclopentane ring (D). In steroids, the phenanthrene ring system is completely saturated (hydrogenated) and is thus referred as perhydrophenanthrene.

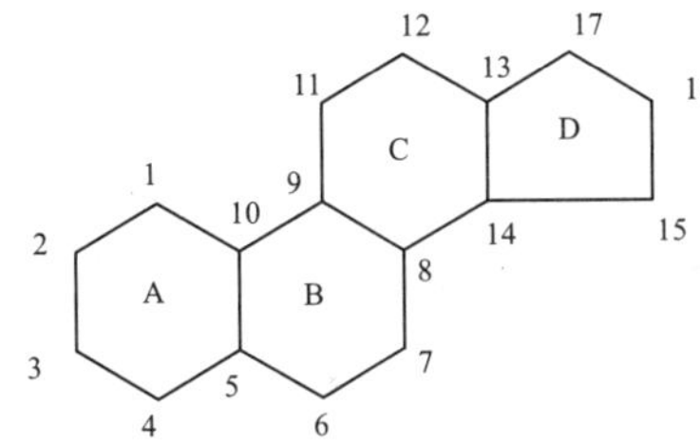

Cyclopentano perhydrophenanthrene

Steroids vary by the functional groups attached to this four-ring core and by the oxidation state of the rings. The numbering of the carbon atoms begins with the carbons of the phenanthrene ring A. In addition, they contain two angular - CH_3 (C_{18} and C_{19}) groups attached to C_{10} and C_{13} respectively. There is a presence of oxygen containing functional group at C_3 followed by with or without carbon side chain at C_{17}.

The ring A, B and C are 6-membered, whereas ring D is 5-membered. The ring A/B system occur either *cis* or *trans*. The rings B/C is *trans* fused only in natural steroids, whereas rings C/D are always *trans* fused. The ring system in which the A, B ring junction is *trans* become the 5α series; and the ring system in which the A, B ring junction is *cis* becomes the 5β series. In the compound six centers of asymmetry exist (C_5, C_8, C_9, C_{10}, C_{13} and C_{14}), thus $2^6 = 64$ stereoisomeric forms are theoretically possible. Depending upon the number of substitutions, the center of asymmetry goes up to eight and the number of stereoisomers to 256.

The three-dimensional shapes of the rings in the steroid skeleton are not planar. The cyclohexane ring experienced flip or puckered conformation and ring D exists in a half-chair conformation. The steroids are rigid in structures because of *trans* fused-ring system, and these rings must be diequatorial to each other. The diequatorial *trans* fusion between rings A and B results in the hydrogen atom at position 5 to be above the plain and 5α designation used for this hydrogen. The axial-equatorial *cis* fusion between rings A and B result in the hydrogen atom at position 5 to be below the plain and designated as 5β.

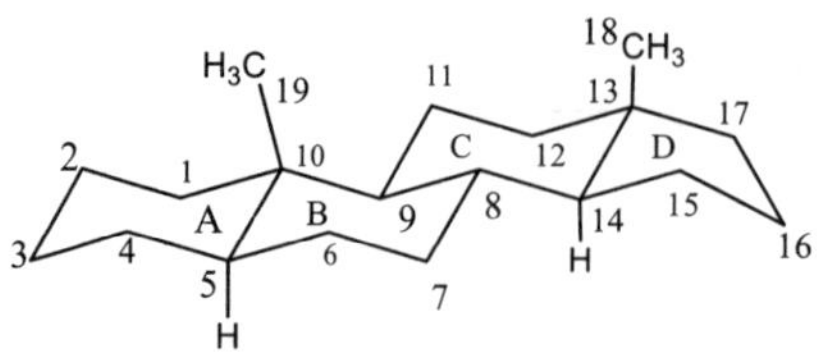

All ring junction are trans

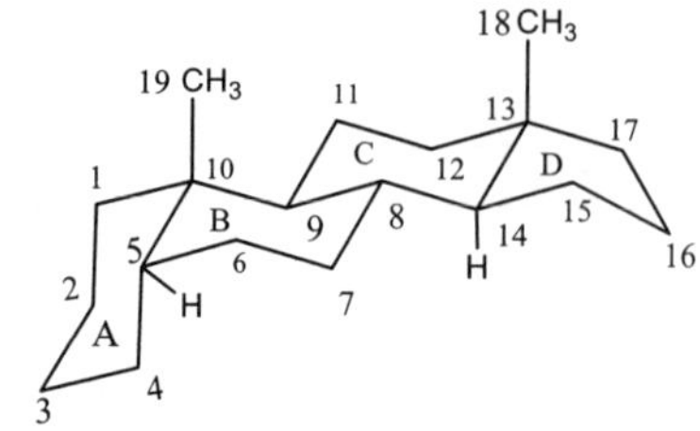

A/B ring junction is cis B/C and C/D trans

1.2 Nomenclature

Early days trivial names used for steroid hormones such as cholesterol, cortisol, progesterone, testosterone, oestradiol etc., As more steroid molecules were being discovered or synthesized, more systematic method for naming steroid was needed (IUPAC). The systematic names for steroids are based on the steroid hydrocarbon system, begins by selection of the stem name based closely those for other organic compounds, with special features to accommodate the stereo chemical aspects.

The basic steroidal ring cyclopentano perhydrophenanthrene contains 17 carbon atoms and the numbering starts at the A ring, continues at B, C and then D ring. Methyl groups at angular positions 13 and 10 are given numbers 18 and 19, the numbering then continues in the side chain. The numbers are used to indicate the positions at which substituents or multiple bonds are attached in individual compounds.

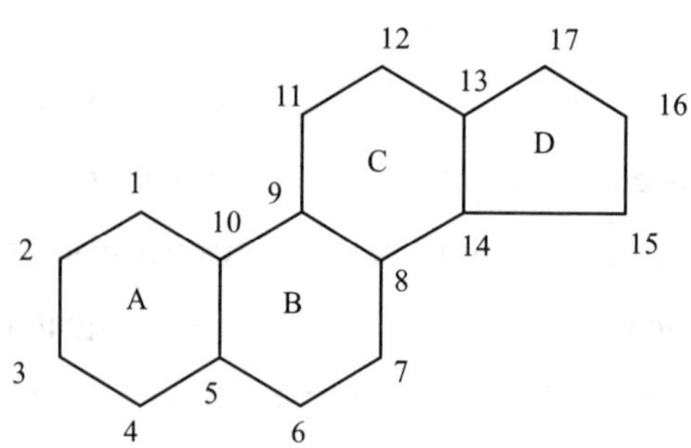

Cyclopentano perhydrophenanthrene

Most steroid compounds are derived from the following six basic hydrocarbons

Parent hydrocarbon	Number of Carbon	Structure
Gonanes	Contains 17 carbon atoms Parent tetracyclic hydrocarbon without methyl groups at C-10 and C-13 and no substitution at C-17	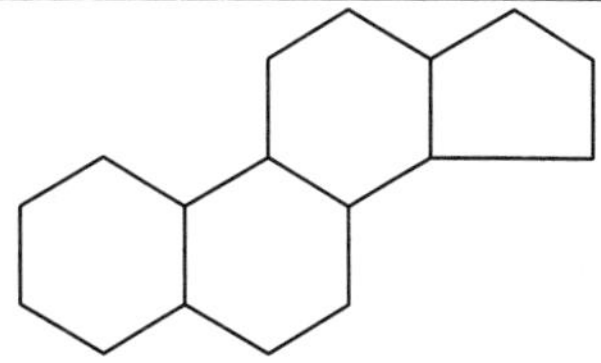
Androstane	Contains 19 carbon atom and methyl groups at angular positions C-10 and C-13. Present in male sex hormone - Testosterone.	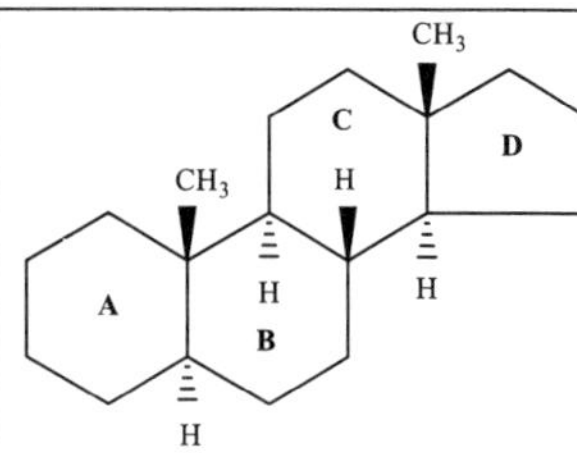 5α - Androstane
Oestrane	Contains 18 carbon atom methyl groups at angular positions 13. Present in oestrogens	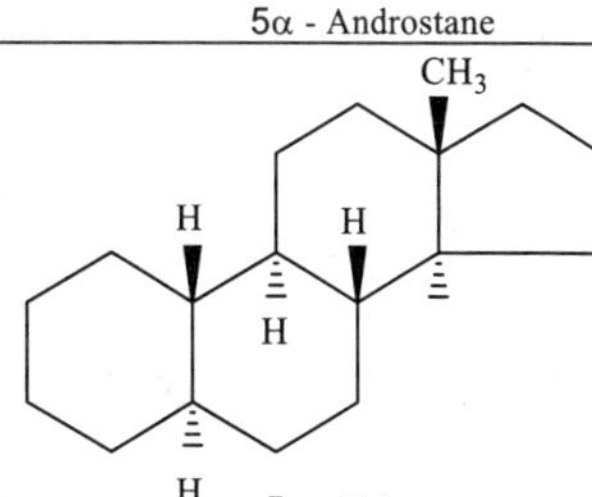 5α - Estrane
Pregnane	Contains 21 carbon atom and methyl groups at C-10 and C-13, with a side chain at C-17 up to C-21. Present in progesterone and adrenocortical hormones	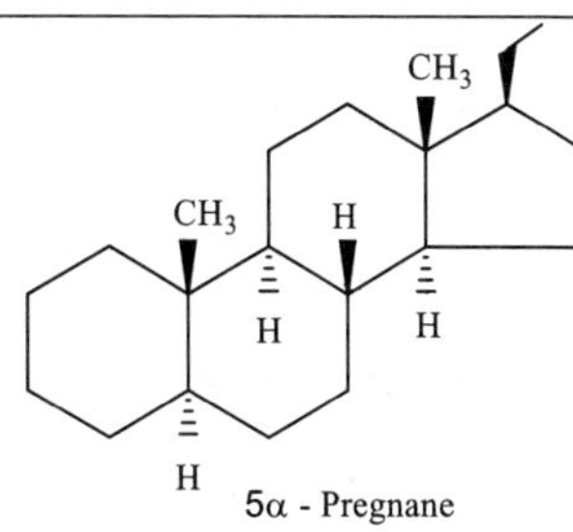 5α - Pregnane

Cholane	Contains 24 carbon atom and methyl groups at C-10 and C-13, with a side chain at C-17 up to carbon chain 24. Found mainly in cholic alcohols and acids	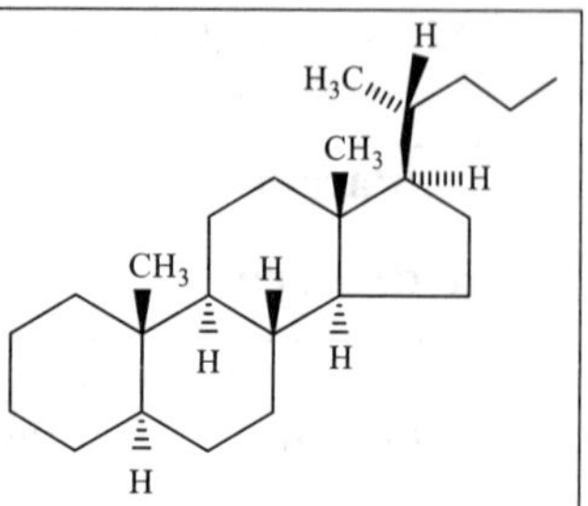
Cholestane	Contains 27 carbon atom Foundation of sterols and their derivatives	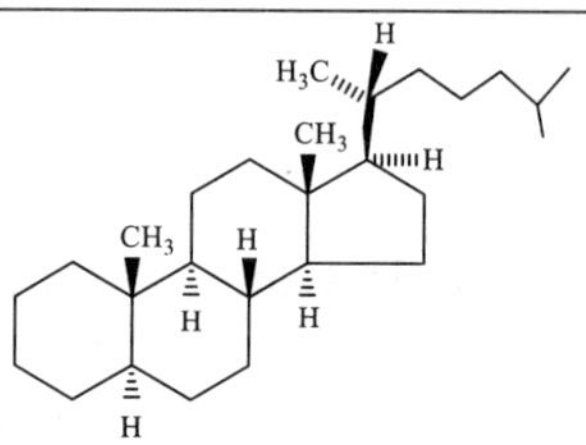

1.3 **Procedure for Naming a Steroid**

- ✓ Appropriate hydrocarbon is selected based upon the carbon skeleton
- ✓ A group or hydrogen at particular carbon, shown by thick line, indicated above the plane of the nucleus and is designated as beta (β) configuration and shown by dotted line is below the plane and is termed as alpha (α).
- ✓ If the configuration of the substituent is unknown its bond to the nucleus is drawn as a wavy line and this is indicated by ξ(xi) in the name.
- ✓ Wherever possible, the name of the steroid should specify stereo chemical configuration. The configuration of the H at C_5 is always indicated in the name.
- ✓ Any unsaturation is indicated by replacing the terminal 'ane' by 'ene', 'diene', 'triene', 'yne', etc., according to the number of double (or triple) bonds present. Substituent groups are indicated either in suffix or in prefix form, as in general organic nomenclature.

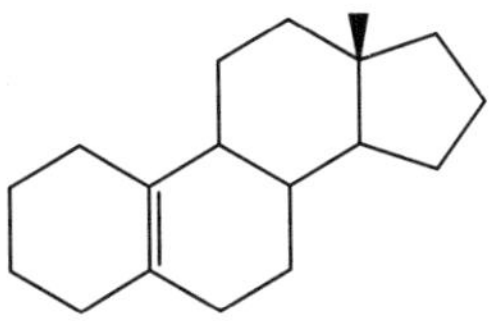

Estr - 5(10) - ene

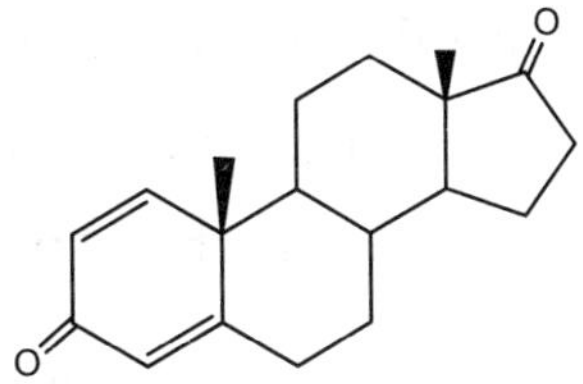

Androsta - 1, 4 - diene - 3, 17 -dione

- ✓ If the double bond is not present between sequentially numbered carbons in such cases both the carbons are indicated in the name.
- ✓ When a methyl group missing from the side chain indicated neither by the prefix "nor" with the number of the carbon atom, which has disappeared.

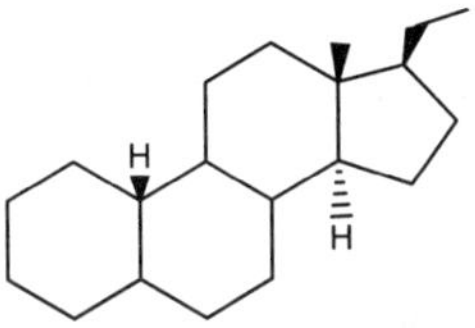

19 - Nor - 5α - pregnane

- ✓ The symbol Δ is often used to designate a C = C bond in a sterol. If the double bond is between C_4 and C_5 the compound is referred as Δ^4 steroid. If the double bond is between the position C_5 and C_{10}, then the compound is designated as $\Delta^{5(10)}$ steroid.
- ✓ When a ring has contracted, indicated by prefixes 'nor'. The prefix homo-similarly indicates added or enlarged carbon atoms proceeded by a small capital letter indicating the ring affected. Eg. 17a-homo-5α-androstane

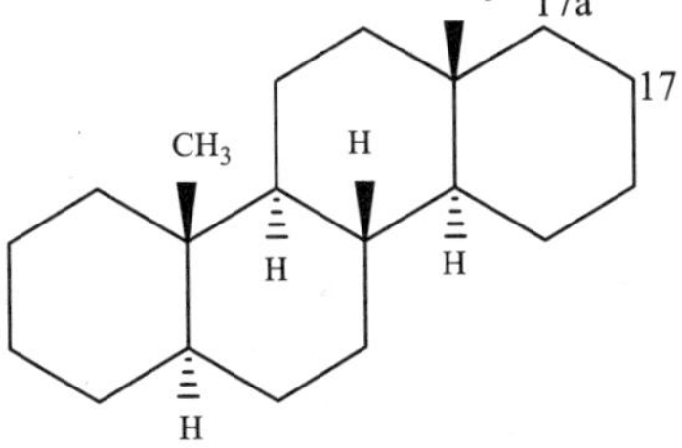

17a - Homo - 5α - Androstane

- ✓ When ring-fission has occurred, this is indicated by the numbers showing the position of the bond broken, followed by prefix 'seco'. The prefix 'cyclo' is used to indicate a three- membered ring.

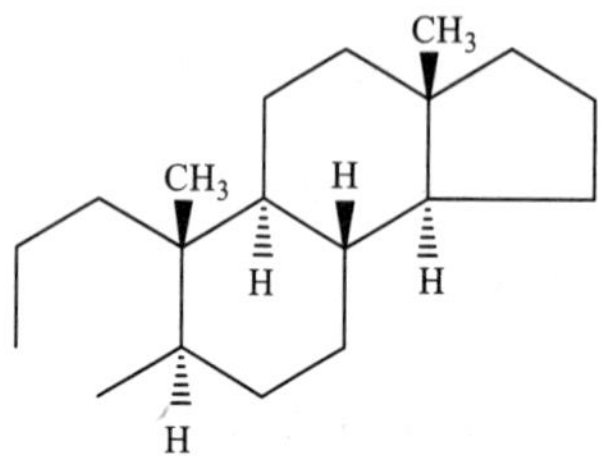

3, 4 - Seco - 5α - androstane

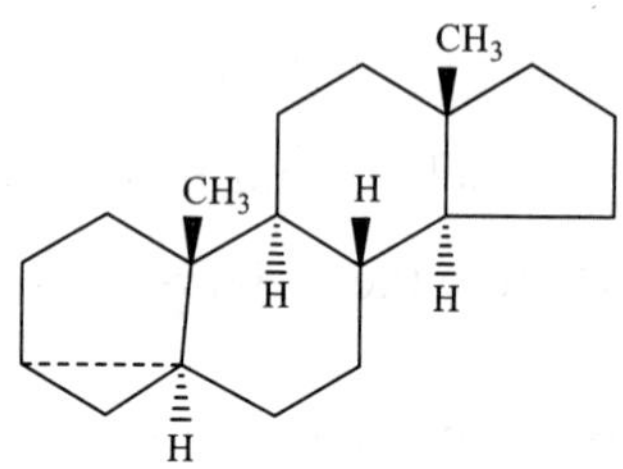

3α, 5α - Cycloandrostane

- ✓ Compounds which are derived from 5α-chloestane belongs to the allo-series, whereas compounds derived from 5β-cholestane (coprostane) belongs to the normal series.

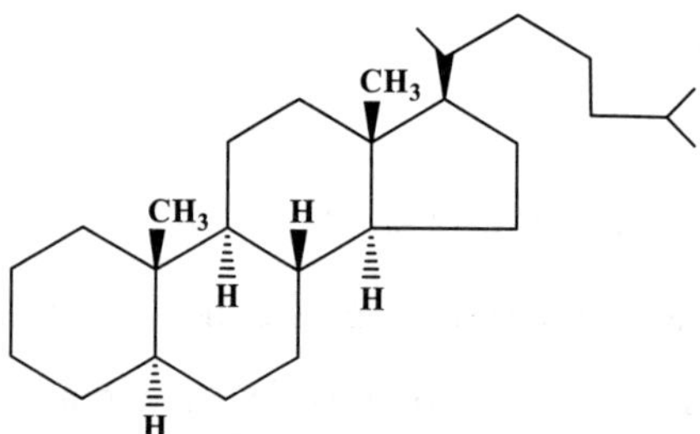

5α - Cholestane

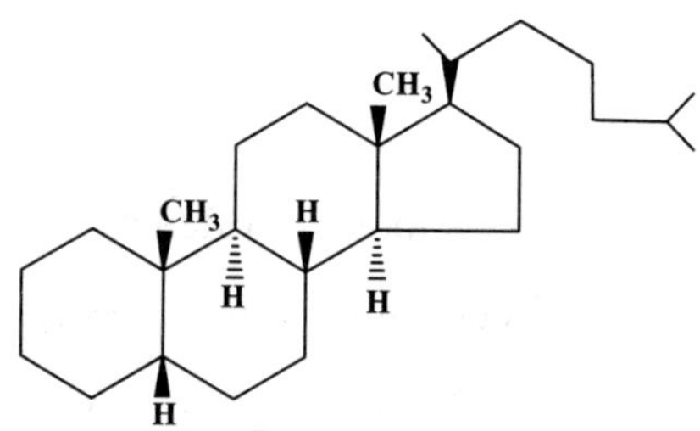

5β - Cholestane

- ✓ When the carbon skeleton of a steroid carbon atom is replaced by a hetero atom [O, N, S] the replacement system of nomenclature is used with steroid names and numbering.

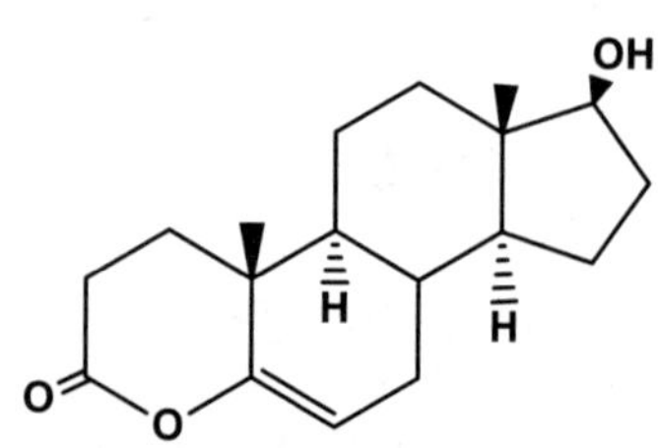

17β - Hydroxy - 4 - oxaandrost - 5 - en - 3 - one

1.4 Biosynthesis and Metabolism

Steroidal hormones are biosynthesized from cholesterol in mammals. Cholesterol is stored in endocrine tissue and is converted into pregnenolone serves as a precursor in the formation of adrenocorticoids and sex hormones. The main routes of biosynthesis are depicted in Fig.10.1

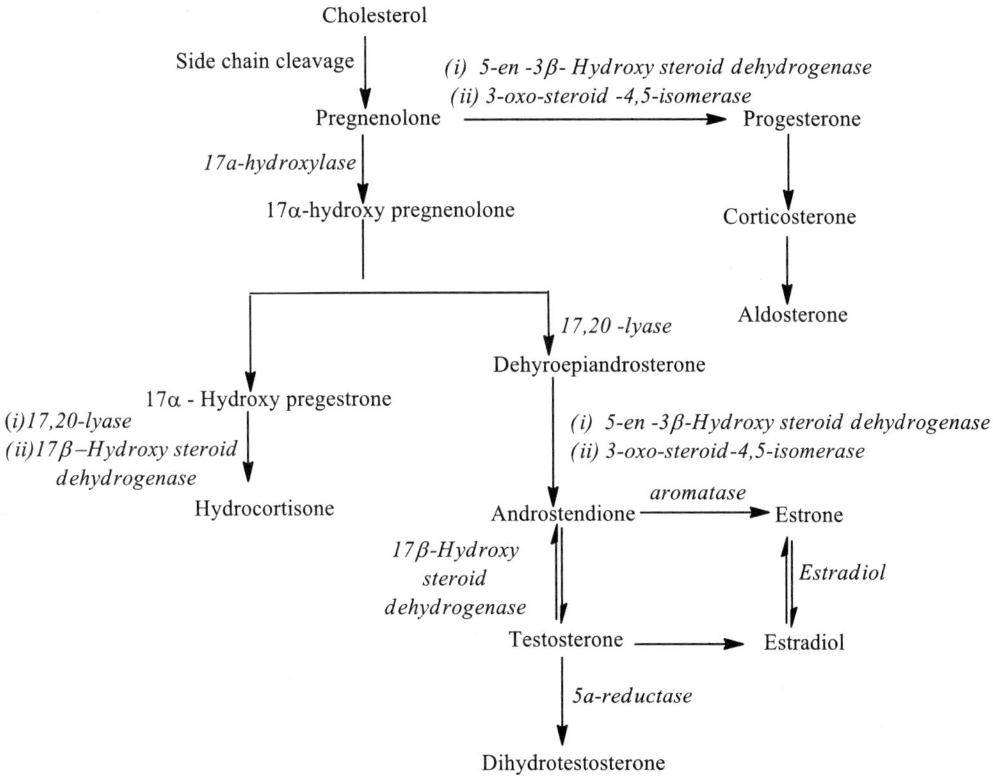

Fig. 10.1 Biosynthesis of Steroids

Enzymes which produce steroidal hormones from cholesterol are located in mitochondria and endoplasmic reticulum. Steroids are lipid soluble and thus are freely permeable to membranes so are not stored in cells. Because of their lipophilic properties, free steroid molecules are only sparingly soluble in water so carried in the blood as either in a conjugated form, i.e. linked to a hydrophilic moiety (eg. as sulfate or glucuronide derivatives) or bound to proteins (non-covalent, reversible binding). Corticosteroid binding globulin carries cortisol.

Sex steroid binding globulin carries Testosterone and Oestradiol. In some cases, a steroid is secreted by one cell and is converted to the active steroid by the target cell (androgen is secreted by the gonad and converted into oestrogen in the brain). Steroid hormone synthesis is largely regulated at the initial steps of cholesterol mobilization and transport into the mitochondrial matrix for conversion to pregnenolone. In the body, the fate of pregnenolone is tissue-specific: in the zona fasciculata of the adrenal cortex it is converted to cortisol, in the zona glomerulosa to aldosterone and in the gonads to testosterone and then to Oestrone and Oestradiol. The main site of peripheral steroid inactivation and catabolism is the liver, but some catabolic activity also occurs in the kidneys. Inactive hormones are mainly eliminated as urinary (mostly conjugated) metabolites.

1.5 Mechanism of Action

The steroidal hormones (S) act on the target cell to regulate gene expression and protein biosynthesis via the formation of steroid-receptor complex. In addition to structural similarity adrenocorticoids, oestrogen, progestin and androgens share a common mode of action. Steroidal hormones travel in the blood and attach to the protein carriers (P). When it reaches the target cell, they enter in the cell through diffusion.

Some steroidal hormones bind to the specific protein in the cytoplasm and move as a hormone receptor complex into the nucleus. Others travel directly into the nucleus before encountering their receptor (R) protein or bind to the binding sites in the nucleus. When the hormone binds to the receptor, a characteristic series of event occurs:

- ❖ The binding initiates conformational changes in the receptor known as receptor activation. The major consequence of receptor activation is that the receptor becomes competent to bind DNA.
- ❖ Activated receptor binds to particular region of the DNA, referred as "hormone responsive element" and promotes hormone responsive gene.
- ❖ This stimulates transcription from the gene to produce mRNA.
- ❖ Finally, the elevated level of mRNA leads to an increase in protein synthesis in endoplasmic reticulum. These proteins include enzymes, receptors and secreted

factors that results in steroidal hormone response regulating cell function, growth etc.,

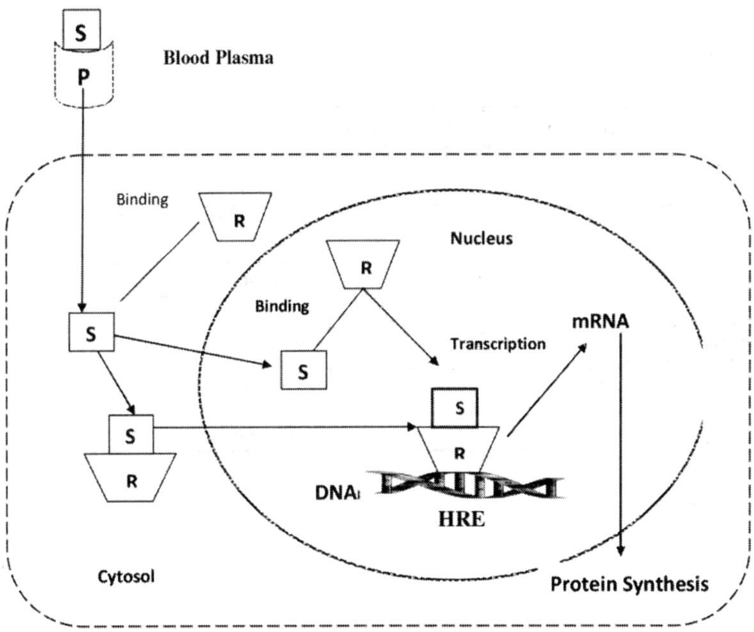

S-Steroidal Hormone**; R-** Receptor; **HRE**-Hormone Responsive Element

Fig. 10.2 Diagrammatic Representation of Mechanism of Action of Steroidal Hormones

2. SEX HORMONES

Sex hormones are usually classified as follows

i) Androgens (Male sex hormones)

ii) Oestrogens (Female or Follicular hormones)

iii) Gestogens (The corpus luteum hormones)

2.1 Androgens

The first androgen Androsterone was isolated from the male urine. The second and third such hormones from the males were Dehydroepiandrosterone and Testosterone respectively. Androgen comprises a group of steroids which produces biological effects of primary and secondary sex characteristics. Androgens are male sex hormones produced mainly by the testes, ovary and adrenal cortex. They possess potent anabolic and androgenic properties. Testosterone is 10 times more potent than Androsterone.

2.1.1 Classification

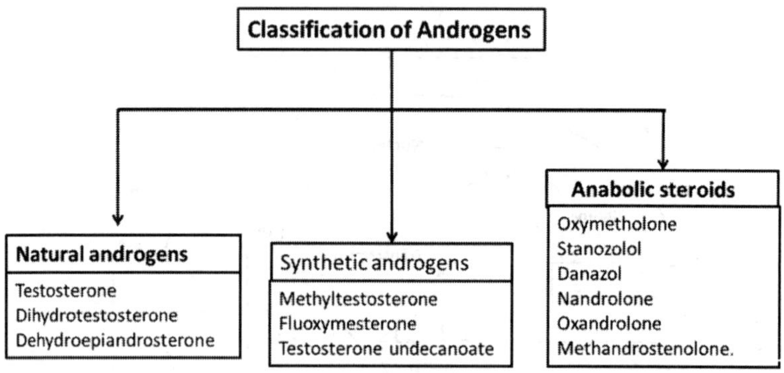

2.1.1.1 Natural Androgens

A. Testosterone

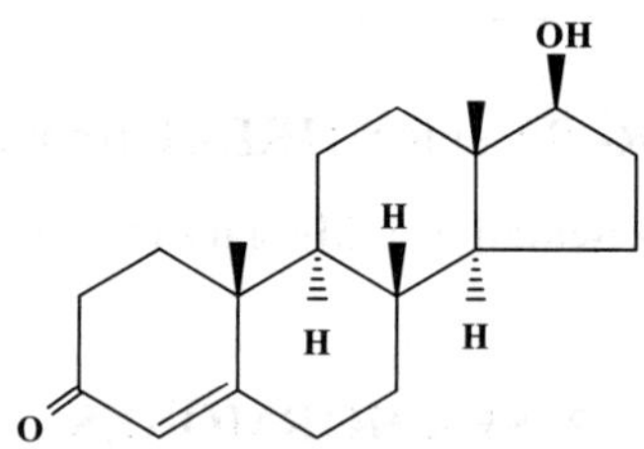

Testosterone

17β - Hydroxy - 4 - androsten - 3 - one

It is naturally occurring androgens in men. It is available in a transdermal delivery system, a gel formulation and as implantable pellets. It is only weakly active orally, but its esters exhibit prolonged or delayed action, thus reducing the frequency of injection. This may be due to slow hydrolysis to limited solubility or to slow uptake from the site of injection.

Mechanism of action: Testosterone and its active metabolite dihydrotestosterone (DHT) antagonize the androgen receptor to develop masculine sex organs including the prostate, seminal vesicles, penis and scrotum. Antagonism of the androgen receptor is also responsible for the development of secondary sexual characteristics including facial and body hair, enlargement of the larynx, thickening of the vocal cords and changes in muscle and fat distribution.

Use: Testosterone and structurally related androgens are used to treat male hypogonadism, Klinefelter syndrome (a chromosomal abnormalities resulting in testicular dysfunction), aplastic anemia and as antiandrogens.

2.1.1.2 Anabolic Steroids

Anabolic steroidal hormones are synthetic substances that are related to male sex hormones. They have the same mechanism of action within the body. Anabolic steroidal hormones stimulate the production of protein, which is used to build muscle. They also lead to an increase in the production of Testosterone. In addition to its role in the development of reproductive system organs and sex characteristics, testosterone is also critical in the development of lean muscle mass. Additionally, anabolic steroid hormones promote the release of growth hormone, which stimulates skeletal growth.

A. Nandrolone (Durabolin)

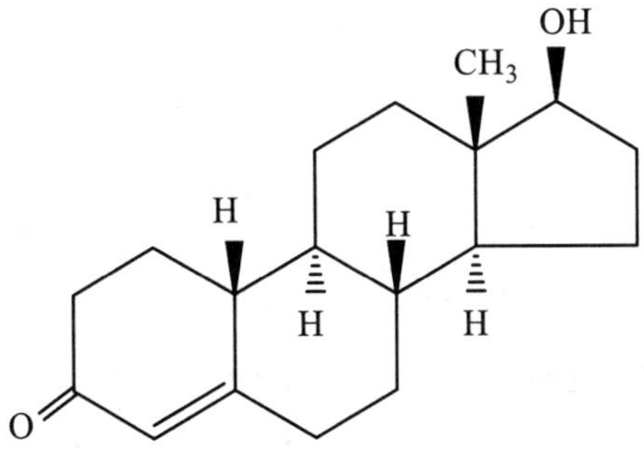

17β - Hydroxy - 4 - oestren - 3 - one

It is also known as 19-nortestosterone. It is an androgen and anabolic steroid used in the form of esters decanoate and phenyl propionate.

Mechanism of action: It is an androgen receptor agonist. The drug bound to the receptor complexes which allow it to enter the nucleus and bind directly to specific nucleotide sequences of the chromosomal DNA. The areas of binding are called hormone response elements (HREs) and influence transcriptional activity of certain genes, producing the androgen effects.

Use: It is mainly used in the treatment of chronic wasting diseases and osteoporosis. It has long duration of action.

2.2 Gestogens (Corpus Luteum Hormones)

The natural gestogen is Progesterone, which is secreted mainly by corpus luteum portion of the ovary. Small amount is also secreted by the testes in the male and the adrenal cortex in both the sexes and large amounts are secreted by the placenta. eg. Progesterone

2.2.1 Classification

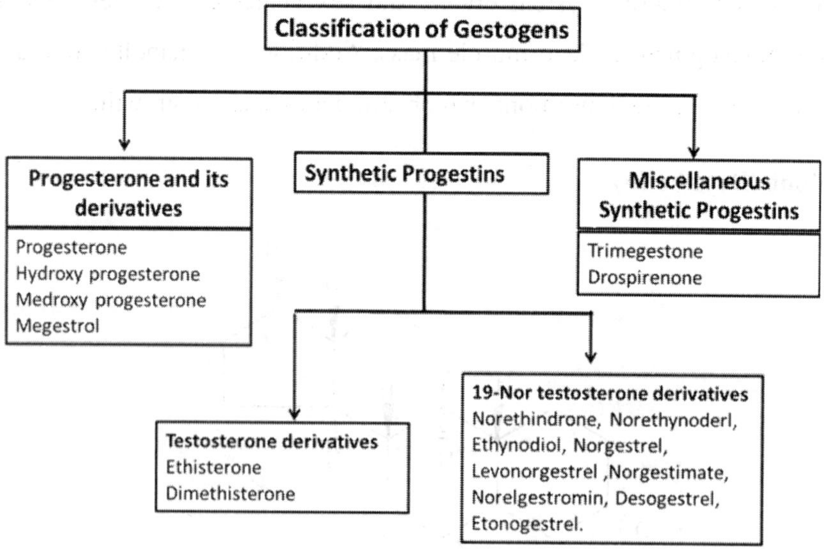

2.2.1.1 Progesterone and its Derivatives

A. Progesterone (Ongest, Algest)

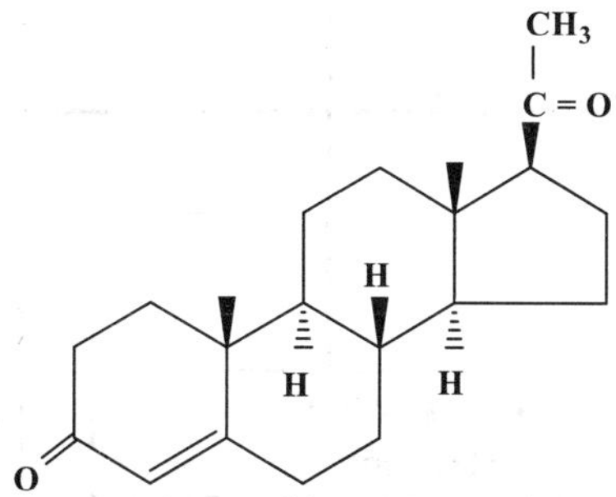

4 - Pregnen - 3, 20 - dione

Progesterone is the main hormone of corpus luteum and placenta. Progestogens are necessary for certain changes which occur in the uterus and vagina during menstrual cycle, for the development of mammary tissue and for the maintenance of pregnancy. It is not active orally.

Mechanism of action: Progesterone binds to nuclear/steroid hormone receptor and undergoes conformational changes with progesterone response element that regulates transcriptase.

Use: It is used in the treatment of functional uterine bleeding. It is given along with oestrogen in menstrual disorder and also given in the treatment of neoplasm of the breast and the endometrium.

2.3 Oestrogens

Oestrogens are a steroid hormone associated with the female reproductive organs and are responsible for the development of female sexual characteristics. It is also needed for maintenance of pregnancy and has anabolic effect on protein metabolism and water retention. Oestrogens also help to regulate the menstrual cycle, controlling the growth of the uterine lining during the first part of the cycle.

2.3.1 Classification

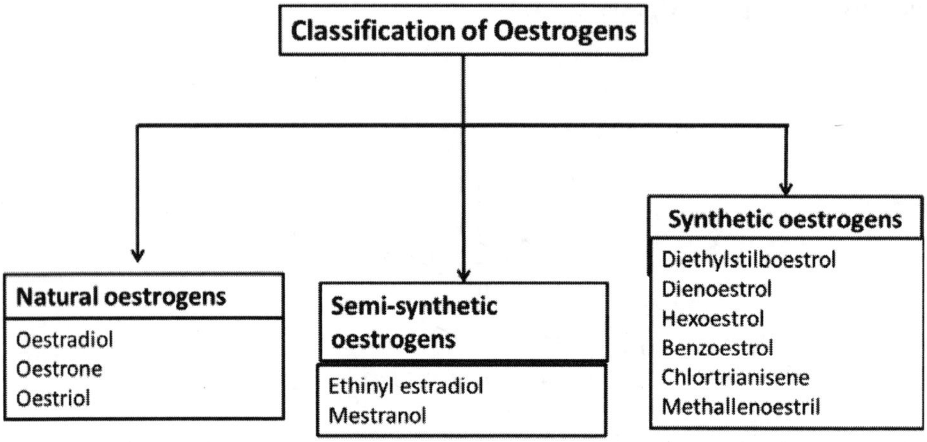

2.3.1.1 Natural Oestrogens

There are three major natural oestrogens namely Oestrone, Oestradiol and Oestriol are secreted by ovary. Oestradiol is also known as 17β-oestradiol. It is a principle oestrogen in premenopausal women. Oestrone and Oestriol are metabolite of Oestradiol *in vivo*. Oestrone is about 1/3rd as active as Oestradiol and Oestriol is about 1/6th as active as Oestradiol. Oestrone is circulating hormone after menopause and Oestriol is significant during pregnancy because it is produced by placenta.

Oestrone	Oestriol	Oestradiol (Vagifem)
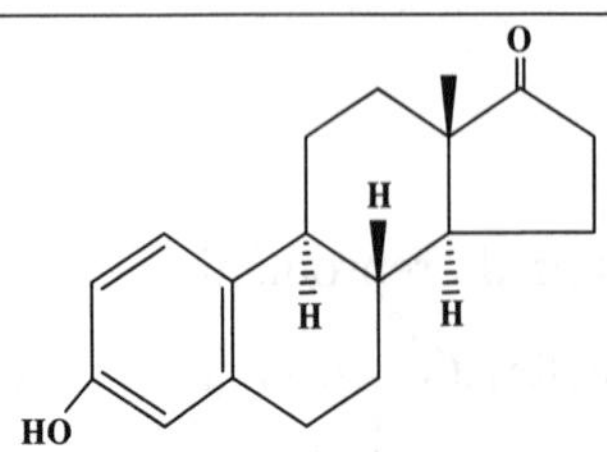 3 - Hydroxyoestra - 1, 3, 5 - (10) - trien - 17 - one	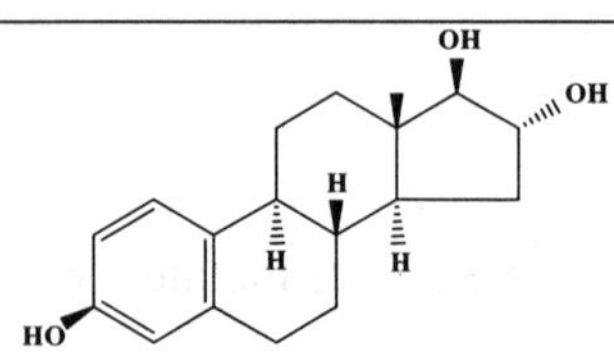 3β, 16α, 17β - Trihydroxy oestra - 1, 3, 5 - (10) - triene	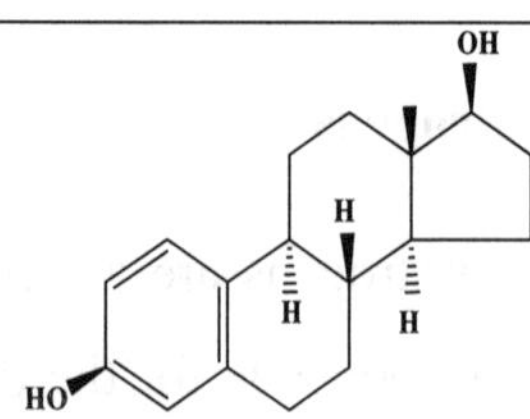 3β,17β - Dihydroxy oestra - 1, 3, 5 - (10) - triene
It is mainly used for the treatment of delayed onset of puberty and management of	Used in gynecological problems, such as endometriosis, fibroids	Used to regulate the maintenance of female

menopausal syndrome.	and cancers that occur in females, particularly endometrial cancer.	sex organs.

Mechanism of action: Oestrone diffuses through the cell membrane and binds to and subsequently activates the nuclear oestrogen receptor. The activated hormone-receptor complex binds to the oestrogen response element on the DNA and promotes the transcription of target genes involved in the functioning of the female reproductive system and secondary sex characteristics.

Use: It is used in hormonal contraceptive, hormone replacement therapy and to treat gender dysphoria in transgender women.

2.3.1.2 Synthetic Oestrogens

A. Diethylstilboestrol (Estril)

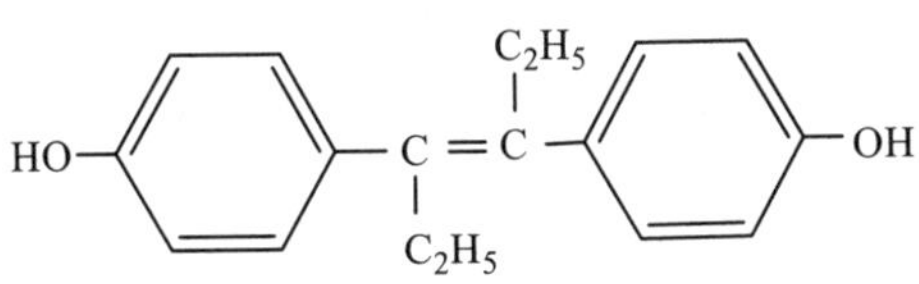

3, 4 - (Di - p - hydroxy phenyl) - 3 - hexene

Diethylstilbestrol is also known as Stilbestrol. It exists in *cis* and *trans* form. *Trans* form is highly estrogenic active than *cis* form. It can also be given orally. It possess similar activity as that of Oestradiol or other natural oestrogens. When compare the structure of Stilbestrol with natural oestrogens, Oestradiol with ring B and C open and a 6-carbon ring D. The distance between the two Stilboestrol phenolic - OH group has the same as that of C_3 - OH or C_{17} - OH distance of Oestradiol. Therefore, they could both fit the same receptor. The - OH to - OH distance in Stilbestrol is actually 12.1A°, whereas 10.9A° in Oestradiol.

Mechanism of action: It works via a steroidal hormone mechanism and a potent full agonist of both of the oestrogen receptors.

Use: It is used for the treatment of prostatic carcinoma. It is a synthetic non-steroidal oestrogen used in the treatment of menopausal and postmenopausal disorders.

3. DRUGS FOR ERECTILE DYSFUNCTION

3.1 Introduction

Erectile dysfunction is defined as persistent difficulty in achieving and maintaining an erection sufficient to have sex. Causes for erectile dysfunction are usually medical but also may be psychological. Organic causes are usually the result of an underlying medical condition affecting the blood vessels or nerves supplying the penis. Numerous prescription drugs, recreational drugs, alcohol and smoking causes erectile dysfunction.

A. Sildenafil (Viagra)

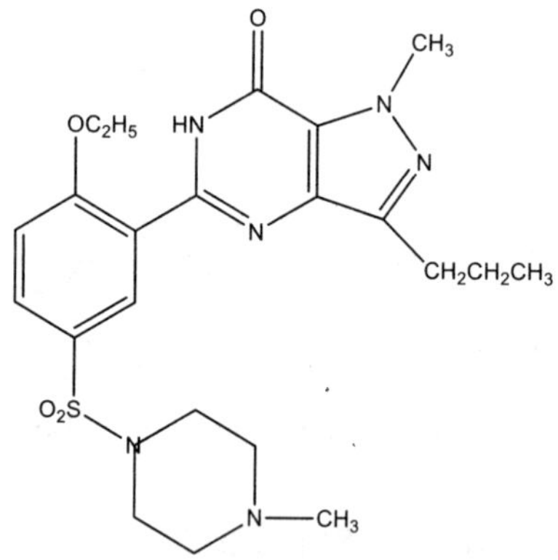

5 -{2 - Ethoxy - 5 - [(4 - methyl piperazin -1- yl) sulfonyl] phenyl} - 1 - methyl - 3 - propyl - 1H, 4H, 7H - pyrazolo [4, 3 - d] pyrimidin -7 - one

Mechanism of action: The physiological mechanism responsible for the erection of the penis involves the release of nitric oxide (NO) in the corpus cavernosum during sexual stimulation. Nitric oxide then activates the enzyme *guanylate cyclase,* which results in increased levels of cyclic guanosine monophosphate (cGMP), producing smooth muscle relaxation in the corpus cavernosum and allowing inflow of blood. Sildenafil is a potent and selective inhibitor of cGMP specific *phosphodiesterase* type-5 (PDE5) in the corpus cavernosum. Inhibition of cGMP degradation results in prolonged muscle relaxation, vasodilation and prolong penile erection.

Use: It is used for the treatment of erectile dysfunction and pulmonary arterial hypertension (PAH).

B. Tadalafil (Cialis)

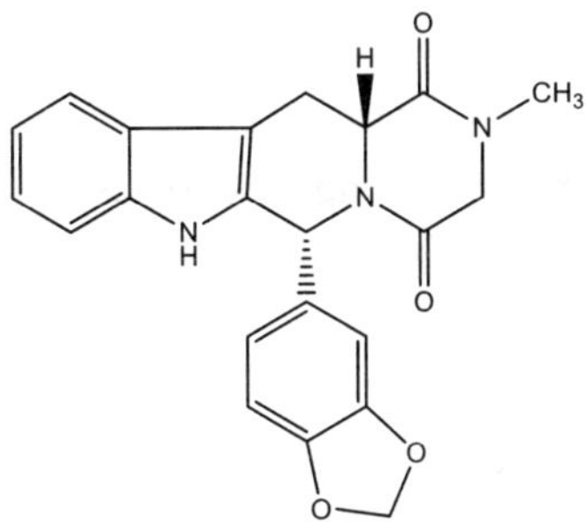

(2R, 8R) - 2 - (1, 3 - Benzodioxol - 5 - yl) - 6 - methyl - 3, 6, 17 - triazatetracyclo [8.7.0.03,8.011,16] heptadeca - 1(10), 11, 13, 15 - tetraene - 4, 7 - dione

It is a carboline based compound having pyrazino-pyrido indole nucleus

Mechanism of action: It selectively inhibits the cyclic guanosine monophosphate (cGMP) specific type-5 *phosphodiesterase* (PDE-5) mediated degradation of cGMP, which is found in the smooth muscle of the corpus cavernosa and corpus spongiosum of the penis. Inhibition of cGMP degradation results in prolonged muscle relaxation, vasodilation and prolong penile erection.

Use: It is an orally administered drug used to treat male erectile dysfunction (impotence) and also used for the treatment of pulmonary arterial hypertension.

4. ORAL CONTRACEPTIVES

4.1 Introduction

Oral contraceptives are medicines taken by mouth to prevent pregnancy. They are also known as pill, OCs or birth control pills. They contain synthetic forms of two hormones produced naturally in the body. These hormones oestrogen and progestin regulate the female menstrual cycle. Some types of oral contraceptives use only progestational hormones, but most use a combination of oestrogen and progestin. Birth control pills do not completely protect a woman from getting sexually transmitted diseases. Contraceptive medications available in various forms such as pills, injections, topical patches and slow release system (vaginal rings, skin implants and contraceptive infused intrauterine devices)

4.2 Type of contraceptives

Oral contraceptives fall into the following categories:

a) Steroidal contraceptives

i) Combination pill

ii) Progestin only pill or mini pill

b) Non-steroidal contraceptives eg. Ormeloxifene

4.2.1 Steroidal contraceptives

4.2.1.1 Combination Pill

It contains combination of oestrogen and progestin. The oestrogen compound either Ethinyloestradiol or Mestranol suppress the follicle stimulating hormone (FSH) release. This prevents the formation of follicle during follicular phase of menstrual cycle. The progestin component (eg. Norethindrone, Norgestimate, Desogestrel, Norgestrel, Levonorgestrel) suppresses the luteinizing hormone (LH) and block ovulation. The combination tablet suppresses the production of FSH and/or LH and prevents ovulation. This process is similar to natural inhibition of ovulation during pregnancy.

Several types of combination birth control pills exist including monophasic pills, biphasic pills, triphasic pills and 91-day cycle pills.

- Monophasic combination pills: The monophasic combination of progestin and oestrogen contains the same amount of drug in each active tablet. The higher Oestrogen/Progesterone ratio early in the cycle develops endometrium. Endometrial effect that prevents implantation of the embryo in the uterus.

The multiphasic formulation more closely mimics the natural changes in both the hormone concentrations that occur throughout the menstrual cycle. The variation in oestrogen and progestin level in multiphasic combinations prevents the incident of spotting (break throughout bleeding) associated with monophasic combination.

- Biphasic pills contain 2 different progesterone doses. The progesterone dose is increased about halfway through the cycle.
- Triphasic pills gradually increase the dose of progesterone and provides higher dose of oestrogen. Three different increasing pill doses are contained in each cycle.
- Post coital morning after pill- Postcoital or emergency contraception is used to prevent unwanted pregnancy after unprotected sexual intercourse (Levonorgestrel emergency contraceptive pill)

4.2.1.2 Progestin only Pill or Mini Pill

The mini pill contains either Norethindrone or Norgestrel. The progestin only pill is given for those patients with contraindications to exogenous oestrogen (eg. smoking or high blood pressure) for old women to whom fertility is diminished or for a lactating woman who already experiencing prolactin-induced ovulation suppression.

A. Mifepristone (Mifeprex)

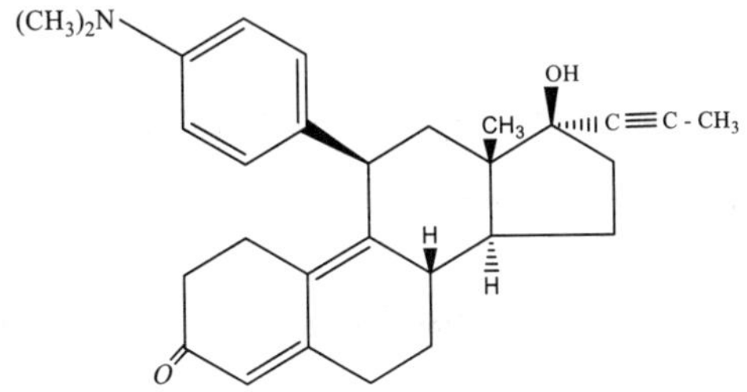

11ß - [p - (Dimethyl amino) phenyl] - 17ß - hydroxy - 17 - (1- propynyl) estra - 4, 9 - dien - 3 - one

Mifepristone also known as RU-486, is a steroidal antiprogestogen, as well as an anti-glucocorticoid.

Mechanism of action: The anti-progestational activity of Mifepristone results from competitive interaction with progesterone at progesterone-receptor sites. It inhibits the activity of endogenous or exogenous progesterone result in termination of pregnancy.

Use: It is used to treat abortion and Cushing's syndrome.

B. Norgestrel (Ovrette, Ovral)

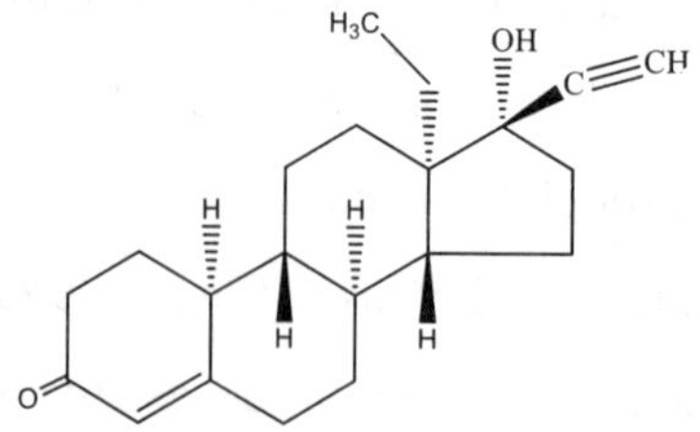

17β - Ethynyl -17α - hydroxy - 18α - homoestr - 4 - en - 3 - one

It is often referred as "mini-pill" because it does not contain any oestrogen. Norgestrel (a form of progestin) prevents pregnancy by making vaginal fluid thicker to help prevent sperm from reaching an egg (fertilization) and changing the lining of the uterus (womb) to prevent attachment of a fertilized egg. It is composed of a racemic mixture of two stereoisomers, Dextronorgestrel and Levonorgestrel. However, only the levorotary enantiomer (Levonorgestrel) is biologically active.

Mechanism of action: It binds to the progesterone and oestrogen receptors within the female reproductive tract, the mammary gland, the hypothalamus and the pituitary will slow the frequency of release of gonadotropin releasing hormone (GnRH) from the hypothalamus and blunt the pre-ovulatory LH (luteinizing hormone). Loss of the LH inhibits ovulation and thereby prevents pregnancy.

Use: It is a synthetic steroidal progestin used in combination with Ethinyl oestradiol for oral contraception.

C. Levonorgestrel (Falessa)

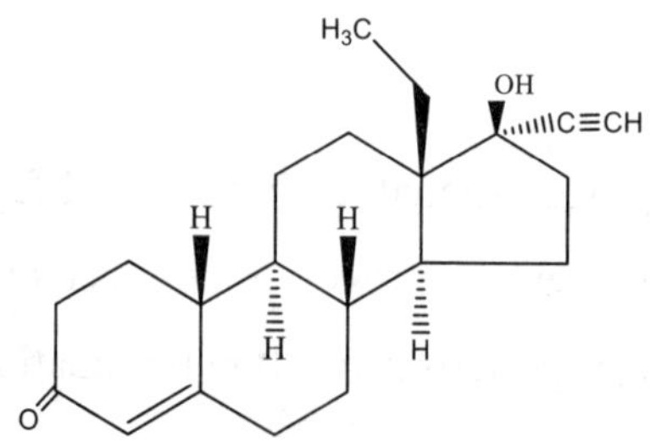

17α - Ethynyl -17β - hydroxy - 18β - homoestr - 4 - en - 3 - one

It is a synthetic progestogen similar to Progesterone used in contraception and hormone therapy. Also known as Plan B, it is used as a single agent in emergency contraception and as a hormonal contraceptive released from an intrauterine device, commonly referred as an IUD. It is the $C_{13}\beta$- or levorotatory stereoisomer and enantiopure form of Norgestrel, the $C_{13}\alpha$- or dextrorotatory isomer being inactive.

Mechanism of action: It suppresses gonadotropins, inhibiting ovulation. Specifically, it binds to progesterone and androgen receptors and slowdown the release of gonadotropin-releasing hormone (GnRH) from hypothalamus. This process results in suppression of the normal physiological luteinizing hormone (LH) surge that precedes ovulation. It inhibits the rupture of follicles and viable egg release from the ovaries. Levonorgestrel has been proven to be more effective when administered before ovulation.

Use: Used as a single agent emergency contraceptive pill. It is used in various hormone-releasing intrauterine devices for long-term contraception. It is prescribed in combination with oestradiol as hormone therapy during menopause to manage vasomotor symptoms and to prevent osteoporosis.

5. ADRENAL CORTICAL HORMONES

5.1 Introduction

The adrenal gland, located below kidney is a flat and cap like structure. The cortex (shell) of the gland synthesizes steroid hormone known as adrenocorticoids, whereas the medulla (inner core) of the gland secrets catecholamines. The adrenocorticoids include glucocorticoids and mineralocorticoids. Glucocorticoids regulate carbohydrates, proteins and lipid metabolism. Mineralocorticoid regulates salt balance and water retention. The decreased secretion of steroidal hormone by the adrenal cortex results in Addison's disease (named after Thomas Addison) characterized by weakness, anorexia, hypotension, vomiting, hyper pigmentation of skin and mental depression.

Cushing's syndrome is hyperadrenalism, increased secretion of adrenocorticotropin hormone due to pituitary carcinoma. The inability of adrenal cortex to carry 17α-hydroxylation from cholesterol during the biosynthesis of the hormone, results in increased aldosterone level, characterized by polyurea, alkalosis, hypernatremia and hypertension is known as Conn's syndrome.

The most important steroidal hormones are produced by adrenal cortex are Aldosterone a primary mineralocorticoid in humans and Hydrocortisone a primary glucocorticoid in humans. Adrenal cortex hormones are classified into two classes.

i) Glucocorticoids

ii) Mineralocorticoids

5.2 Glucocorticoids

Glucocorticoids are secreted by adrenal cortex, that affect the carbohydrate and protein metabolism and which favor lipolysis called glucocorticoids. They exert a regulatory influence on lymphocytes, erythrocytes and eosinophils of the blood. Glucocorticoids are used in the treatment of collagen vascular diseases like rheumatoid arthritis, disseminated lupus erythematous and dermatomyositis. They are also used topically, orally and parenterally in the treatment of anti-inflammatory conditions. They also provide relief from symptoms of allergy like hay fever, dermatitis, eczema etc.,

5.2.1 Classification

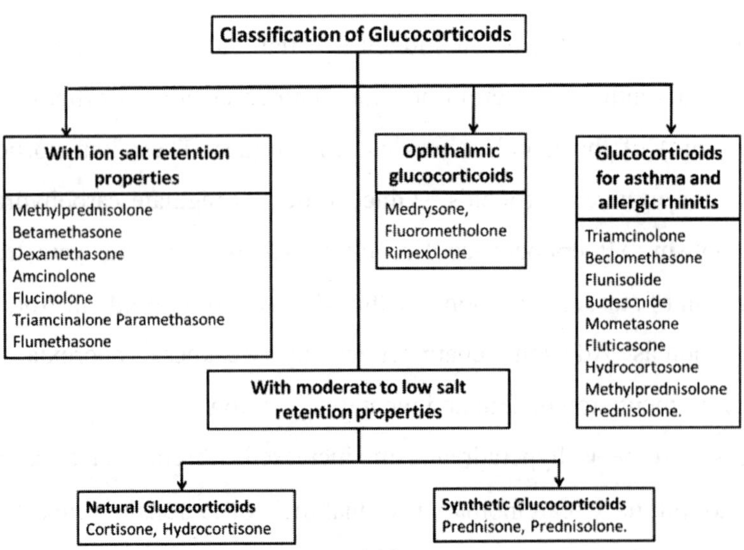

Mechanism of action: It is as a corticosteroid hormone receptor agonist a member of the nuclear receptor family of ligand-activated transcription factors. It binds to intracellular glucocorticoid receptors and suppresses inflammatory and immune responses by inhibiting synthesis of inflammatory response mediators, such as cytokines, interleukins and prostaglandins.

5.2.1.1 Natural Glucocorticoids

A. Cortisone (Corlin)

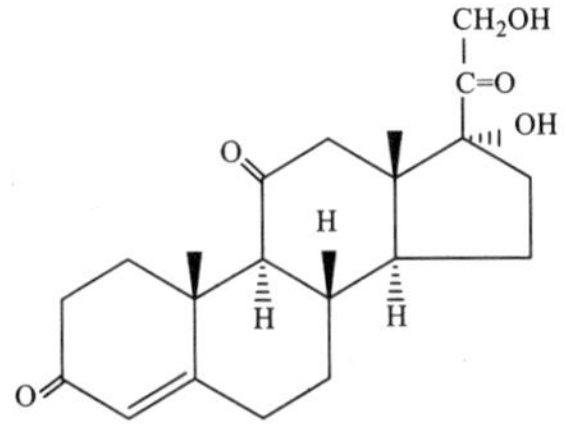

17α,21-Dihydroxy-4-pregnen-3,11,20-trione

Cortisone is naturally occurring corticosteroid with good systemic anti-inflammatory activity and low-to-moderate salt retention activity. It is official as Cortisone acetate. Cortisone is the inactive precursor molecule of the active hormone Cortisol, which is the hydroxylation product of cortisone by *11β-steroid dehydrogenase* which increases blood pressure, blood sugar levels and suppresses the immune system, so Cortisone is used to treat allergies or inflammation.

Use: It is used in the treatment of collagen diseases, Addison's disease, severe shock, allergic conditions and chronic lymphocytic leukemia.

B. Hydrocortisone (Cort-S, Multicort)

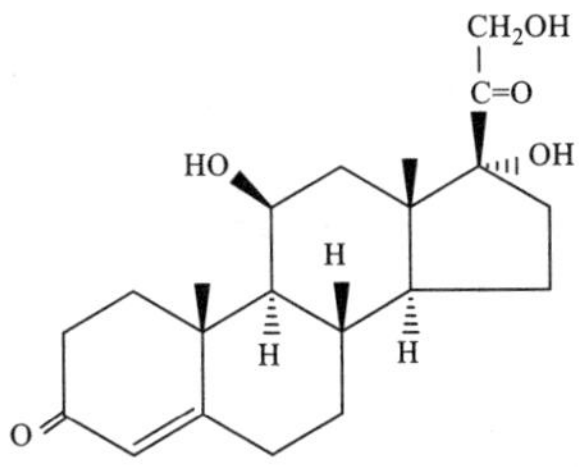

11β, 17α, 21 - Trihydroxy - 4 - pregnen - 3, 20 - dione

Hydrocortisone is the primary natural glucocorticoids in humans. It contains -OH group at C_{11} instead keto group, when compare to the structure of Cortisone.

Use: It is mainly used in hormone replacement therapy, shock, status asthmatics and acute adrenal insufficiency.

5.2.1.2 Synthetic Glucocorticoids

A.Prednisolone (Predone, Predcip)

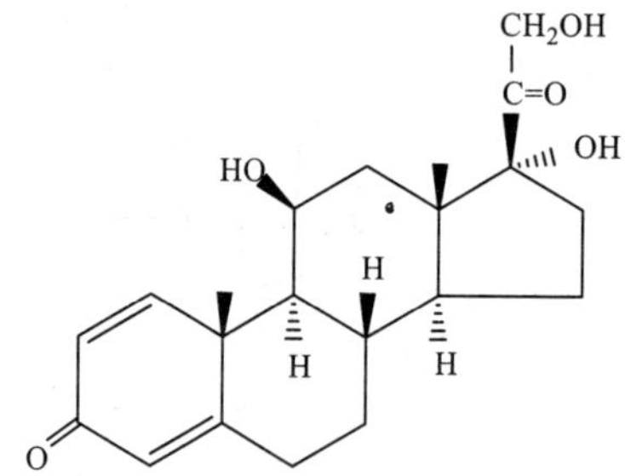

11β, 17α, 21 - Trihydroxy -1,4 - pregnadien - 3,20 -dione

Prednisolone is Δ^1hydrocortisone. It is a corticosteroid drug with predominant glucocorticoid and low mineralocorticoid activity.

Use: It is used for allergic, inflammatory, autoimmune diseases and in malignancies.

5.2.1.3 Fluoro Derivatives

A. Betamethasone (Betnesol, Betnovate)

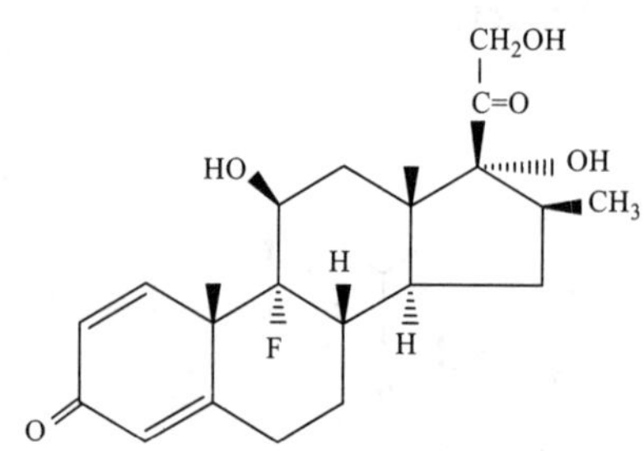

9α -Fluoro - 11β, 17α, 21 - trihydroxy - 16β - methyl - 1,4 - pregnadien - 3,20 - dione

It has increased glucocorticoid and anti-inflammatory activities, but very low mineralocorticoid activity. It is effective with very low dose. It is available as variety of ester derivatives like Betamethason-17-valerate, Betamethason-21-acetate, Betamethason-21-sodium phosphate, Betamethason-17, 21-dipropionate. Unlike other drugs with these effects, it does not cause water retention.

Use: It is used for inflammatory, allergic conditions, also preferred in cerebral edema, skin irritation and flake from eczema. The combination of Betamethasone dipropionate and salicylic acid is used to treat psoriasis.

B. Dexamethasone (Decdan, Decatron, Dexona)

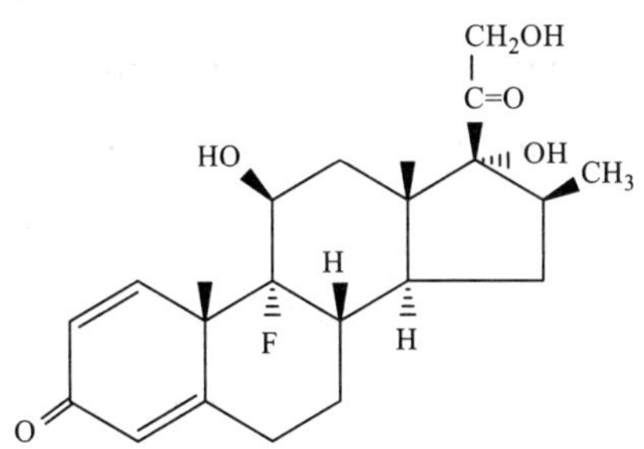

9α - Fluoro - 11β, 17α, 21 - trihydroxy - 16α-methyl -1,4 - pregnadien - 3,20 - dione

Dexamethasone is a 16α-isomer of Betamethasone. It is available as Dexamethasone-21-acetate and Dexamethason-21-sodium phosphate. It possess glucocorticoid activity. Its glucocorticoid potency is about 25 times as that of Cortisone.

Use: It is used for inflammatory, allergic conditions and also preferred in cerebral edema and shock.

THYROID AND ANTITHYROID DRUGS

Chapter 11

1. THYROID DRUGS

1.1 Introduction

The thyroid gland is a large endocrine gland located deep in the neck, close to the uppe portion of trachea. The two major thyroid hormones are thyroxine (T_4) and triiodo thyroxin (T_3), Thyroid hormones are derivatives of the amino acid tyrosine bound covalently to iodine Synthesis of the thyroid hormones requires iodine uptake into the thyroid gland an incorporation into tyrosine residues in the major thyroid protein, thyroglobulin. T_3 is the mos biologically active form of thyroid hormone and exerts its effects by binding to the thyroi hormone receptor. Thyroid hormone is a member of the steroid hormone/thyroid hormon superfamily of nuclear receptors. Thyroxine was first isolated in crystalline form from hydrolysate of thyroid gland by Kendall in 1915.

The primary functions for the thyroid hormones are fetal and post-natal developmen development of the CNS, modulation of cardiac function through regulation of myocardia contraction and relaxation, renal water clearance, gastrointestinal motility, thermal regulatior energy expenditure and regulation of lipid metabolism. The thyroid gland also synthesizes th peptide hormone, calcitonin, from parafollicular C cells. However, human calcitonin has n physiological role in humans but the protein is an important marker for thyroid medullar carcinomas.

1.2 Bio-synthesis of Thyroid Hormone

The formation of thyroid hormones involves the following complex sequences:

- **Active Uptake of Iodide by Follicular Cells:** The first step in the synthesis of thyroid hormone is the uptake of iodide from the blood by the thyroid gland. Dietary iodide is converted into iodide. Iodide uptake is blocked by certain inorganic ions such as thiocyanate and perchlorate.

- **Oxidation of Iodide and Formation of Iodotyrosine:** The iodide undergoes oxidation by a membrane bound enzyme called *thyroid peroxidase.* Once in the gland, the iodide is oxidized to iodine (organification) it bound to tyrosine and form either monoiodotyrosine or di-iodotyrosine.

- **Coupling of Iodotyrosine Residues**: Coupling this two inactive iodotyrosine yields a hormonally active tetra-iodothyronine (T_4 or l-thyroxine) *and* tri-iodothyronine (T_3 or l-thyronine). This reaction is also catalyzed by the same *peroxidase* enzyme. The hormone remains bound to thyroglobulin through peptide link and remain stored in the follicular colloid.

- **Proteolysis of Thyroglobulin and Release of Iodothyronines**: The secretion of thyroid hormone is mediated by the release of proteolytic enzyme from lysosome, which completely breaks down the thyroglobulin into its constituent amino acids, releasing L-Thyroxine and L-Triiodo thyroxine into the circulation. The proteolysis is stimulated by thyroid stimulating hormone (TSH).

Production of thyroid hormone is maintained by secretion of TSH by the pituitary gland, which in turn is regulated by secretion of thyrotropin-releasing hormone (TRH) in the hypothalamus. The stereo chemistry of the thyroid hormones plays an important role in defining the activity of the hormone. The naturally occurring hormones are biosynthesized from L-tyrosine and possess the L-alanine side chain. The L-isomers of T_4 and T_3 are more active than the D-isomers.

1.3 Thyroid Dysfunctions

- **Hypothyroidism**: Deficiency of thyroid hormone results in hypothyroidism. This causes goiter, cretinism and myxedema. An enlarged palpable thyroid gland is referred as goiter. Cretinism, the irreversible clinical entity characterized by defective physical and mental development, appears when thyroid hormone is not available in early childhood for normal bone formation and normal brain growth and differentiation. Myxedema, a condition marked by slowing down of all the metabolic process of the body. Hashimoto's disease is an auto immune condition in which plasma cells, lymphocytes and fibrous tissue attack and destroy the thyroid gland. Hypothyroidism resulting from it requires lifelong treatment with thyroid hormone replacement. Thyroid hormone and dried thyroid glands are used in the treatment of hypothyroidism.

- **Hyperthyroidism:** Excessive secretion of thyroid hormone results in hyperthyroidism. This causes Grave's disease characterized by thyrotoxicosis and ophthalmopathy. The anti-thyroid drugs are employed in the treatment of hyperthyroidism.

1.4 Synthetic Thyroid Hormones

Synthetic, crystalline thyroid hormones are more uniformly absorbed than biological preparations and contain more precisely measured amount of active ingredients in their dosage forms.

A. L - Thyroxine (Thyrox, Eltroxin)

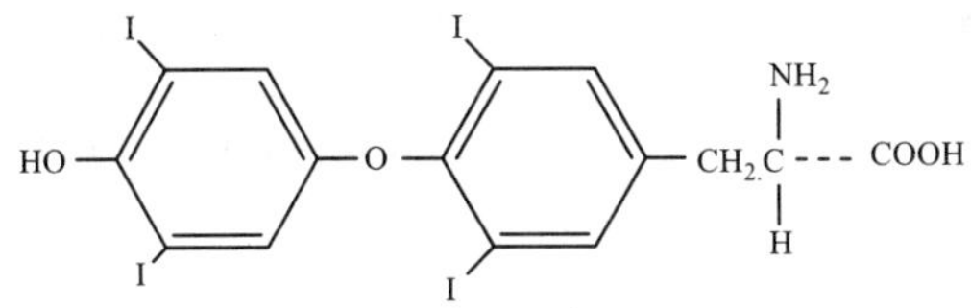

O - (4 - Hydroxy - 3, 5 - diiodophenyl) - 3, 5 - diiodo - L - tyrosine

Oral L-thyroxine is a synthetic hormone that exerts the same physiological effect as endogenous T_4, thereby maintaining normal T_4 levels when a deficiency is present.

Mechanism of action: Levothyroxine is a synthetically prepared *levo* isomer of the thyroid hormone thyroxine (T_4, a tetra-iodinated tyrosine derivative) that acts as a replacement in deficiency syndromes such as hypothyroidism. It replaces endogenous thyroid hormone and then exerts its physiological effects by controlling DNA transcription and protein synthesis.

Use: It is mainly used to treat hypothyroidism.

B. L- Thyronine (T_3, Liothyronine)

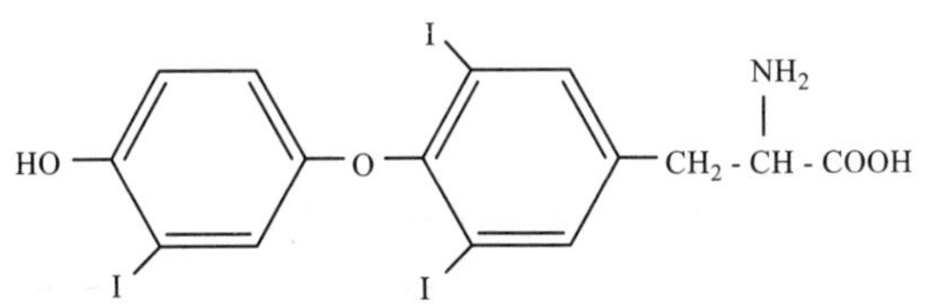

O - (4 - Hydroxy - 3 - iodophenyl) - 3, 5 - diiodo - L - Tyrosine

L-thyronine is the active form of thyroxine which is composed in a basic chemical structure by a tyrosine with bound iodine. L-Thyronine has a rapid onset of action.

Mechanism of action: L-Thyronine replaces endogenous thyroid hormone and then exerts its physiological effects by controlling DNA transcription and protein synthesis. This effect on

DNA is obtained by binding of L-Thyronine to the thyroid receptors attached to DNA. Exogenous liothyronine exerts all the normal effects of the endogenous thyroid T_3 hormone.

Use: It is used in conditions where rapid and short duration of action is required. It is also used to treat hypothyroidism.

2. ANTITHYROID DRUGS

2.1 Introduction

Antithyroid drugs are capable of interfering directly or indirectly with the synthesis, release or action of thyroid hormones and are used to control hyperthyroidism. Hyperthyroidism may be due to Graves' disease, goiter, abnormal secretion of TSH, thyroiditis or excessive iodine intake. The most important group of antithyroid drug is thioamide derivatives and radioactive iodides. By giving a radioactive form of iodine, the thyroid cells which absorb will be damaged or killed. Because iodine is not absorbed by any other cells in the body, there is very little radiation exposure (or side effects) for the rest of the body.

2.2 Classification

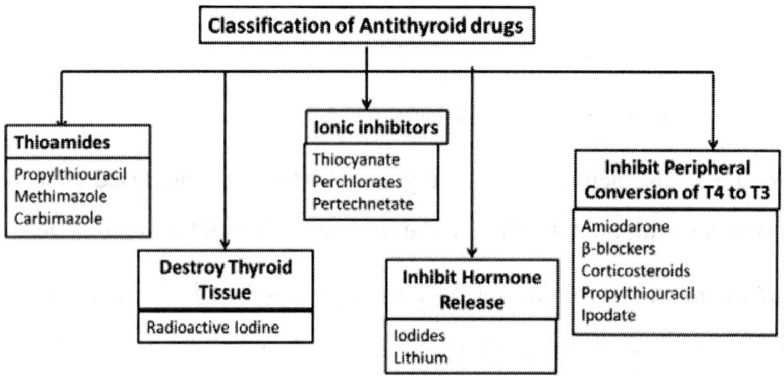

2.2.1 Thioamides

A. Propyl thiouracil (PTU)

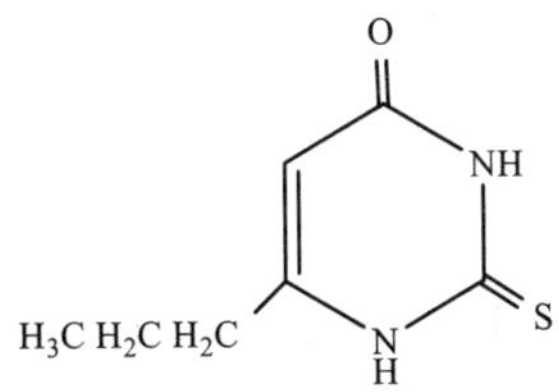

2, 3 - Dihydro - 6 - propyl - 2 - thioxopyrimidin - 4 - one

Mechanism of action: It inhibits the synthesis of thyroxine by inhibiting the enzyme *thyroperoxidase* and prevents the peripheral conversion of thyroxine to tri-iodothyronine.

Use: It is used to control hyperthyroidism in patients with Grave's disease, in preparation of thyroidectomy and as an adjunct to radioiodine therapy.

B. Methimazole (Thiamazole)

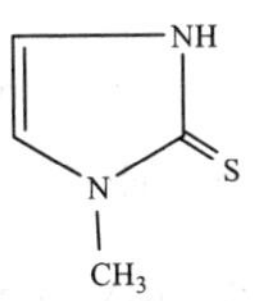

1, 3 - Dihydro -1- methyl - 2H - imidazol - 2 - thione

Mechanism of action: It inhibits the synthesis of thyroxine by inhibiting the enzyme *thyroid peroxidase* and prevents the peripheral conversion of thyroxine to tri-iodothyronine.

Use: It is more potent than Propyl thiouracil and is indicated in the treatment of hyperthyroidism.

Chapter

12

ANTIDIABETIC AGENTS

1. INTRODUCTION

Antidiabetic agents are drugs that stabilize and control blood glucose levels among people with diabetes. It is commonly used to manage diabetes. Deficiency of effective insulin in the body causes a disease called diabetes mellitus (meaning in Greek is excessive thirst) commonly known as diabetes, which alters the metabolism of lipids, carbohydrates and proteins. This results in hyper glycaemia and glycosuria.

There are three main types of diabetes.

i. **Type I diabetes mellitus:** It is formerly known as "insulin-dependent diabetes mellitus (IDDM)" or "juvenile diabetes", occurs when the β-cells of the pancreatic islets of Langerhans are destroyed, such that insulin production is deficient. The loss of β-cell is caused by an autoimmune response.

ii. **Type II diabetes mellitus:** It is formerly known as "non-insulin dependent diabetes mellitus (NIDDM)" is very frequently associated with obesity and insufficient exercise; serum insulin level will be normal or elevated, the problem may be insulin resistance or defect in insulin receptor or post insulin receptor

iii. **Gestational diabetes:** It is a type of diabetes that consists of high blood glucose during pregnancy and is associated with complications to both mother and child.

Antidiabetic agents include

I. Insulin and

II. oral hypoglycaemic agents

2. INSULIN

2.1 Introduction

Insulin is a polypeptide hormone synthesized by β-cells of the islets of Langerhans of the Pancreas (named after Paul Langerhans, 1869) from a precursor proinsulin. Insulin is the primary hormone which is responsible for controlling the storage and utilization of cellular nutrients. It activates the transport system and the intracellular utilization and storage of glucose, amino acids and fatty acids. Insulin inhibits catabolic processes such as the breakdown of glycogen, fat and protein, whereas the overall effect of insulin is hypoglycaemic. Insulin was purified and crystallized by J. J. Abel in 1926.

Insulin consists of two peptide chains A and B, which are connected by two disulphide bonds. The chain A composed of 21 amino acid residue and has one intra-chain disulphide bond; the chain B has 30 amino acids. There are some species-specific differences in the amino acid sequence of insulin (Table 12.1). Porcine insulin differs from human insulin only by the presence of alanine (Ala) instead of threonine as the last amino acid in the chain B and bovine insulin in addition has two more alteration in chain A, the threonine (Thr) and isoleucine (ILE) in 8 and 10 position are replaced by alanine and valine respectively.

Table 12.1 Animal and Human Insulin

Species	**Chain A**		**Chain B 30**
	8	**10**	
Human	Thr	ILE	Thr
Porcine	Thr	ILE	Ala
Bovine	Ala	Val	Ala

Insulin circulates as monomer and only monomers would interact with insulin receptors. The insulin receptor is a large transmembrane glycoprotein composed of four subunits- two identical α-units with M_r of about 130,000 dalton and two β-units with M_r of 95,000 dalton joined together by disulphide bond. The α-subunit is primarily responsible for binding insulin to receptor and β-subunit possesses intrinsic *protein kinase* activity that is stimulated by insulin. The binding of the insulin to the receptor, may result in the generation of a soluble intracellular second messenger that may mediate the activation of enzymes like *pyruvate dehydrogenase* and *glycogen synthetase*. The zinc-associated hexamer is a storage form of insulin in man.

2.2 Production of Insulin

Early commercial insulins were obtained by extraction from bovine or porcine or mixed bovine and porcine pancreas and purified by crystallization. Much of the insulin now produced has amino acid sequence identical to that of human insulin. Presently human insulins are produced by recombinant DNA technology. The recombinant DNA technique for human insulin production involves insertion of the human proinsulin gene into either yeast (*Saccharomyces cerevisiae*) or a non-pathogenic bacterium (*Escherichia coli*) which serve as the production organism. Then human insulin is isolated and purified.

2.3 Insulin Preparation

All insulin preparations are currently generated by recombinant DNA technology. Doses and concentration levels of insulin preparations used are indicated in international units; one international unit of insulin is defined as the bioequivalent of 34.7μg of crystalline insulin. To prolong the duration of action of insulin many attempts have been made by either physical modification like adding protamine or zinc to give crystalline or amorphous form of insulin preparations or altering the amino acid sequence of the analogues. A number of different insulin preparations and analogues are now available. According to duration of action insulin preparations are classified into

- Short-acting insulin
- Intermediate-acting insulin
- Long-acting insulin

(i) Short-acting Insulin

Short acting insulins are used to control the blood sugar at meal times. This insulin is clear solutions at neutral pH and has minor amounts of zinc (for greater stability and shelf life). The insulin molecule generally exists as dimers which can join with zinc ions present in the formulation and form hexamer. After subcutaneous administration insulin monomers are released gradually, so that absorption occurs slowly. The regular human insulin and the rapidly acting insulin preparations are considered as short-acting formulations.

(a) Regular Human Insulin: The water solubility of insulin in body fluids can be altered, so that it is slowly released. The solubility of insulin depends upon particle size (amorphous or crystalline), on zinc content and the nature of the buffer in which it is suspended. Regular insulin is a zinc-insulin crystalline product which has an onset of action of 1/2 hour to 1-hour, peak effect in 2 to 4 hours and duration of action 6 to 8 hours.

(b) Rapid Acting Insulin Analogs: The rapid-acting insulin includes the insulin analogues namely Lispro, Aspart, Glulisine and Techno sphere human insulin. Rapid-acting insulin has an onset of action of 5 to 15 minutes and duration of action that lasts 4 to 6 hours. With all doses, large and small, the onset of action and the time to peak effect is similar.

- Insulin Lispro**:** Proline at location B28 is reversed with the lysine at B29
- Insulin Aspart: Proline B28 replaced by aspartic acid.
- Insulin Glulisine: Asparagine at location B3 is exchanged by lysine and the lysine in location B29 by glutamic acid.
- Techno sphere insulin: It is a dry-powder formulation of recombinant human regular insulin that can be inhaled and absorbed through pulmonary tissue.

(ii) Intermediate-Acting Insulin

Another way of prolonging the action of insulin was, brought by complexing with proteins from which it was slowly released. For example, protamine (basic protein) insulin preparations, prolong the duration of action of insulin. Protamine's are small, highly basic proteins obtained from the sperm of salmon and trout. When added to solutions containing insulin at neutral pH, the protamine molecules bind to insulin and cause it to become insoluble. It is used to control the blood sugar overnight, while fasting and between meals. The two main varieties of Intermediate-acting insulin are Isophane and Lente insulin, which have an onset of insulin effect in 1 to 2 hours and duration of action for 8-12 hours.

(a) Isophane Insulin is a suspension containing equal concentrations of insulin, zinc ions and protamine possess quick onset and short duration than protamine insulin. It is also known as NPH; N indicates neutral pH; P stands for protamine and H for Hagedorn who developed the product. This form of insulin must not be administered through intravenous route. To prevent clogging at the tip of the needle, subcutaneous route is preferred.

(b) Lente Insulin, on the other hand, simply include excess zinc ions in an acetate buffer. This produces fairly insoluble zinc insulin complexes, which can be prepared in two forms:

(c) Ultralente Insulin a crystalline form in which the particles are large and

(d) Semilente an amorphous form with smaller particles that are absorbed more quickly.

(e) Lente Insulin is 70:30 mixtures of Ultra-lente and Semi-lente insulin which has rapid onset of action and intermediate duration of action. Lente insulin is incompatible with Protamine zinc insulin and NPH, because of different buffer system used in the preparation of this insulin. (acetate buffer in Lente insulin; phosphate buffers in Protamine zinc insulin and NPH insulin).

(iii) Long-Acting Insulin

Long acting insulin are absorbed slowly, has a minimal peak effect, and a stable plateau effect that lasts most of the day. Insulin Glargine and Insulin Detemir are long acting insulin analogues, which have an onset of insulin effect in 30 to 60 minutes and duration of action for 12 to 24 hours.

(a) **Insulin Glargine:** It is different from normal insulin, as the asparagine is changed by glycine at amino acid 21 of the insulin A chai, and two arginine residues are added to the carboxyl terminal of the B chain. The pH of this insulin analogue is changed which decreases its solubility. They are also prepared in slightly acidic solution, from which the insulin precipitates when injected at physiological pH is near neutral and leads to more constant absorption.

(b) **Insulin Detemir**: In this threonine at position B30 has been removed and fatty acid myristic acid is attached to the lysine at position 29. The fatty acids bind to albumin in subcutaneous tissue. Albumin is a non-specific binding protein and influence on the rate of absorption of many drugs. Insulin is released slowly and evenly over a long period.

Insulin should be stored in the refrigerator and exposure to extremes temperature lead to loss of insulin effectiveness. Insulin should never be frozen, exposed to direct sunlight or stored in an ambient temperature greater than 30°C.

Use: Insulin is employed for the treatment of virtually all type I and type II diabetic patients. Long term treatment relies on subcutaneous injection.

3. ORAL HYPOGLYCEMIC AGENTS

3.1 Introduction

Oral hypoglycemic agent's lower glucose levels in the blood. They are commonly used in the treatment of diabetes mellitus and given orally. These drugs may also be used with insulin in the management of diabetes mellitus. It is also known as antihyperglycemic agents.

3.2 Classification

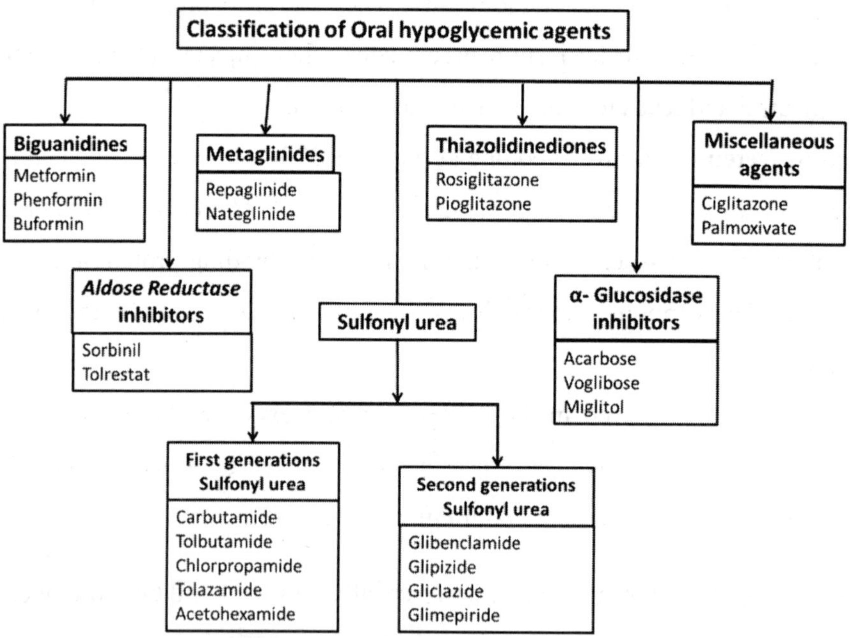

3.2.1 Sulfonyl Ureas

The sulfonyl urea may be represented by the following general structure

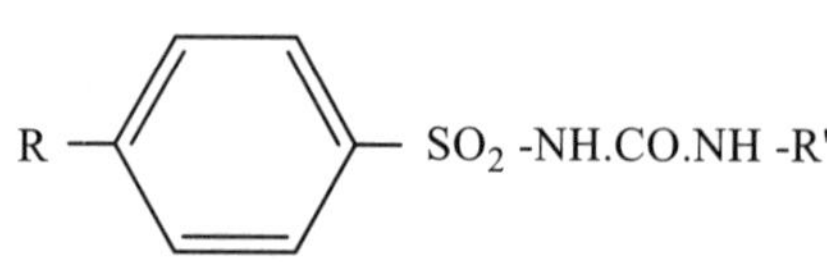

These are urea derivatives with an aryl sulfonyl group in the 1st position and an aliphatic group at the 3rd position. The R group on the aromatic ring primarily influences the duration of action of the compound.

Mechanism of action: The sulfonyl ureas stimulates the release of insulin from the β-cells of pancreas. The ATP dependent potassium channels in β-cell contains sulphonyl urea receptors. Binding with this receptor inhibits these channels and alters the resting potential of the cell. This leads calcium enter into the cell and insulin being secreted. Compared to first generation sulphonyl urea, second generation can be given in much lower dose. They also inhibit the secretion of glucagon.

A. Tolbutamide (Rastinone, Orinase)

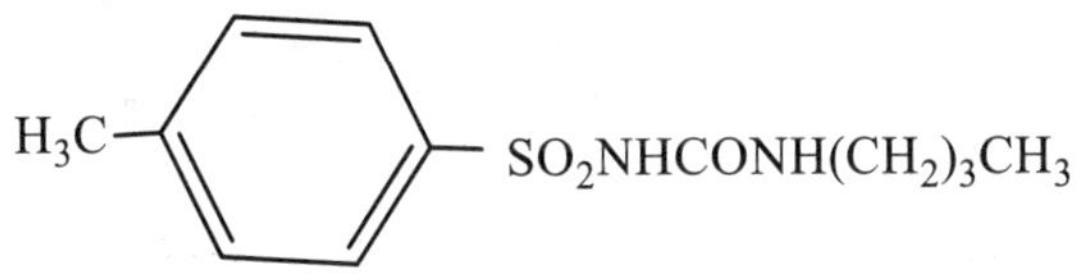

3- Butyl - (p - tolyl sulfonyl) urea

Synthesis

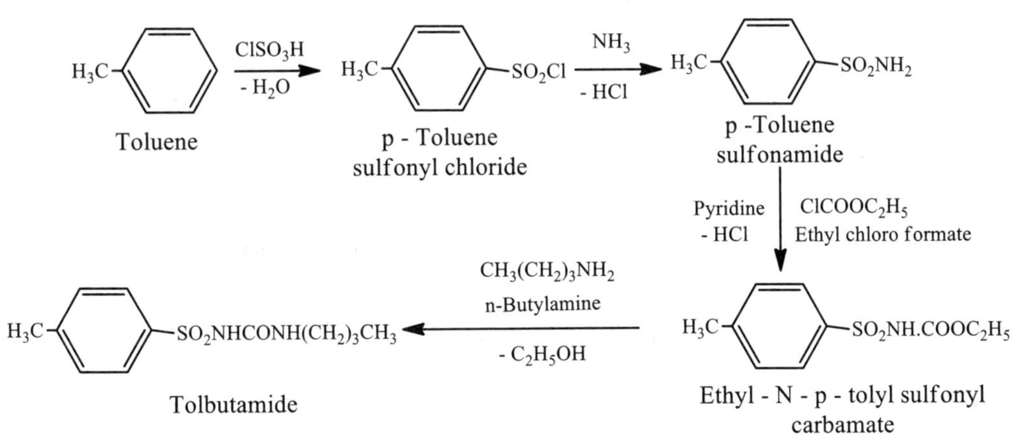

Use: It is an orally active hypoglycemic drug.

B. Chlorpropamide (Copamide, Diabinese)

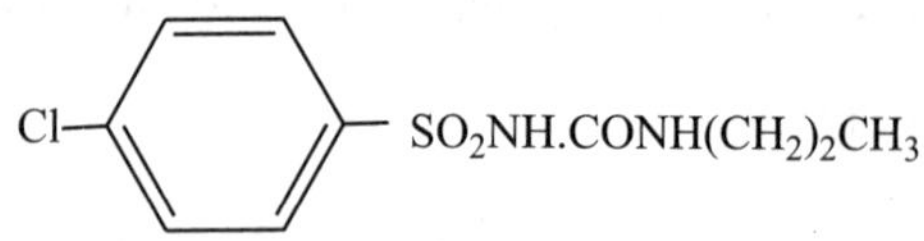

1- [(p - Chloro phenyl) sulfonyl)] - 3 - propylurea

Use: It is an oral hypoglycemic agent used in type II diabetes mellitus.

C. Glipizide (Diaglip, Dibizide)

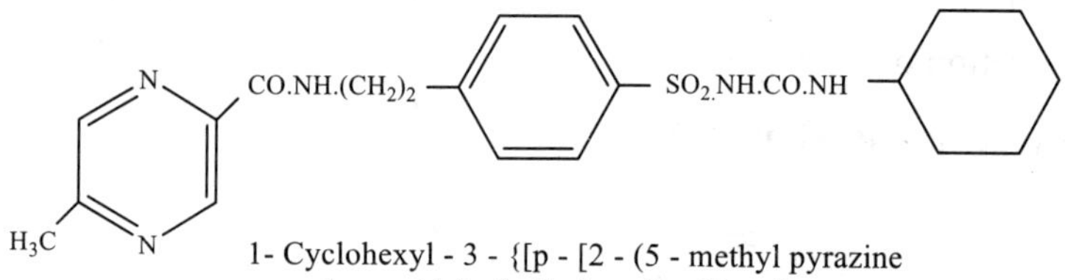

1- Cyclohexyl - 3 - {[p - [2 - (5 - methyl pyrazine carboxamide) ethyl] phenyl] sulfonyl} urea

Use: It is an oral hypoglycemic agent used in type II diabetes mellitus and used together with diet to improve blood sugar control.

D. Glimepiride (Novaride, Glimy)

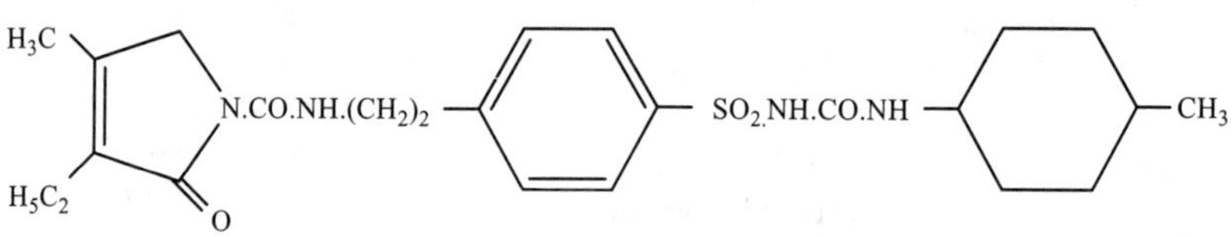

1 - {[p - [2 - (3 - Ethyl - 4 - metnhyl - 2 - oxo - 3 - pyrroline - 1 - carboxamido) ethyl] phenyl] sulfonyl} - 3 - (trans - 4 - methyl cyclohexyl) urea

Use: It is used as an oral hypoglycemic agent in type II diabetes mellitus.

3.2.2 Biguanides

The general chemical structure of biguanide is as follows

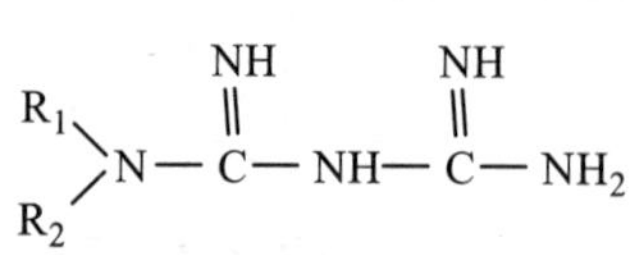

A. Metformin (Glumet, Riomet)

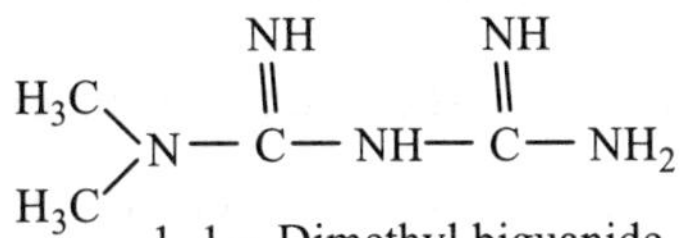

1, 1 - Dimethyl biguanide

Mechanism of action: It decreases hepatic glucose production, intestinal absorption of glucose and improves insulin sensitivity by increasing peripheral glucose uptake and utilization. It activates AMP-activated protein kinase (AMPK), an enzyme that plays an important role in the regulation of glucose metabolism. It also inhibits fat synthesis and leading to fat oxidation, reducing hepatic lipid stores and increasing liver sensitivity to insulin

Use: It is the first drug of choice for the management of type II diabetes mellitus.

3.2.3 Thiazolidinones

Thiazolidinones are a new class of oral antidiabetic agents used for the treatment of NIDDM that enhances insulin sensitivity in peripheral tissues. In addition, they inhibit hepatic gluconeogenesis. These agents normalize glucose metabolism and reduce the amount of insulin needed to achieve glycemic control. They are effective in the presence of insulin.

A. Rosiglitazone (Pioglar, Pioglit)

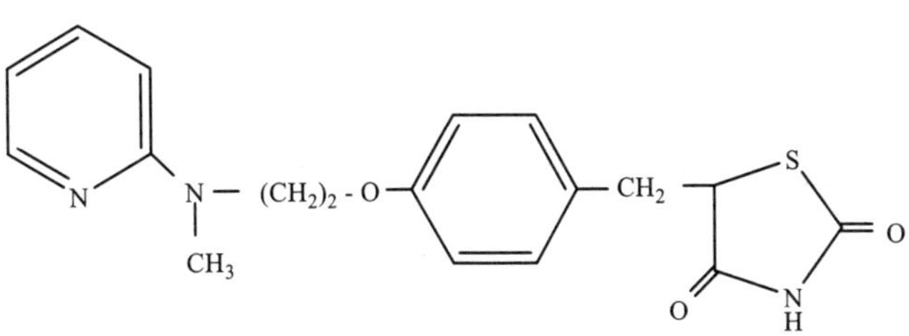

(+) - 5 - {[4 - [2 - Methyl - 2 - pyridinyl amino) ethoxy] phenyl] methyl} - 2, 4 - thiazolidinedione

It possess a single chiral center and is present as a racemate form. Due to rapid interconversion, the enantiomers are functionally indistinguishable.

Mechanism of action: It improves glycaemic control by improving insulin sensitivity. Rosiglitazone bind and activates the peroxisome proliferator-activated receptor-gamma (PPARγ). The PPAR receptor is a key target tissue for insulin action such as adipose tissue, skeletal muscle and liver. Activation of PPARγ nuclear receptors regulates the transcription of insulin-responsive genes involved in the control of glucose production, transport and utilization. In addition, PPARγ-responsive genes also participate in the regulation of fatty acid metabolism.

Use: It is used in the treatment of type-II diabetes mellitus.

B. Pioglitazone (Glizone, Glito)

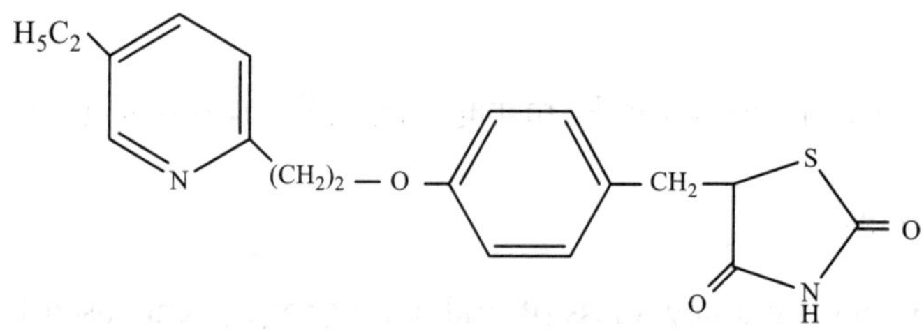

(±) - 5 - {[4 - [2 - (5 - Ethyl - 2 - pyridinyl) ethoxy] phenyl methyl} - 2, 4 - thiazolidinedione

Mechanism of action: It binds and activates the peroxisome proliferator-activated receptor-gamma (PPARγ). Activation of PPARγ nuclear receptors regulates the transcription of insulin-responsive genes involved in the control of glucose production, transport and utilization. In addition, PPARγ-responsive genes also participate in the regulation of fatty acid metabolism.

Use: It is used in the treatment of type-II diabetes mellitus.

3.2.4 Metaglinides

Metaglinides are non-sulfonyl urea oral hypoglycemic agents used in the management of type II diabetes mellitus. They have rapid onset and a short duration of action and these agents induce insulin release from functioning pancreatic β-cells.

A. Repaglinide (Regan, Repa)

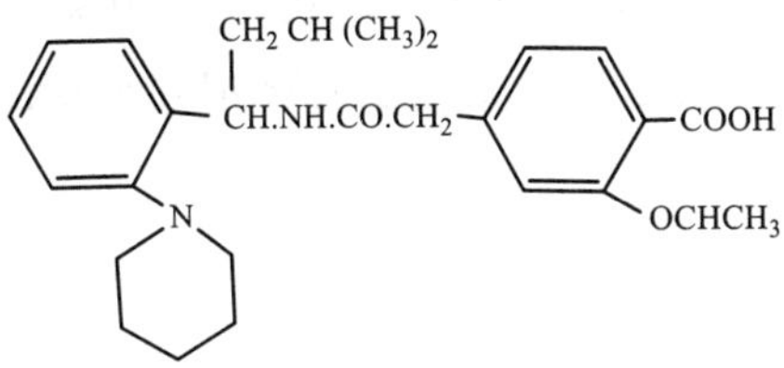

2 - Ethoxy - 4 - [2{[3 - methyl - 1 - [2 - (1 - piperidinyl) phenyl] butyl] amino} - 2 - oxo ethyl] benzoic acid

Mechanism of action: It lowers blood glucose levels by blocking ATP-dependent potassium channels in pancreatic β-cells. The subsequent depolarization of the β-cell opens the calcium channel, producing calcium influx and insulin secretion.

Use: It is used as oral hypoglycemic agent in type-II diabetes mellitus.

B. Nateglinide (Glinate, Nds)

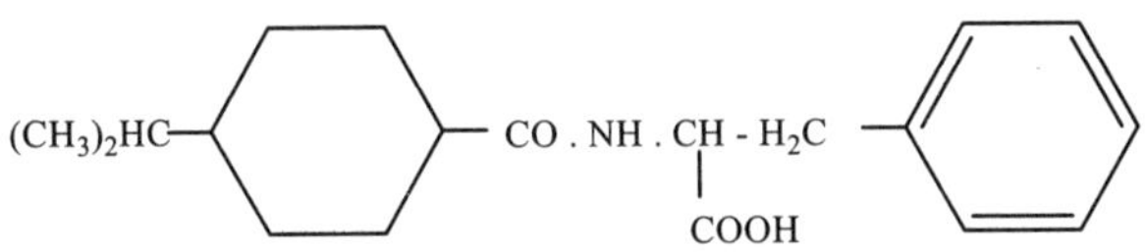

1 - [(4 - Isopropyl) - cyclohexyl carbonyl] -1- phenyl alanine

It is a phenylalanine derivative that lowers blood glucose levels by stimulating insulin secretion from the pancreas.

Mechanism of action: It lowers blood glucose levels by blocking ATP-dependent potassium channels in pancreatic β-cells. The subsequent depolarization of the β-cell opens the calcium channel, producing calcium influx and insulin secretion.

Use: It is used as oral hypoglycemic agent in type-II diabetes mellitus.

3.2.5 *α-Glucosidase* Inhibitors

α-glucosidase inhibitors act as oral antidiabetic drug by inhibiting the *α-glucosidase,* an enzyme present on cells lining the intestine involved in breaking down complex carbohydrates such as starch and glycogen into their monomers. Hence, *α-glucosidase* inhibitor slows and limits the absorption of glucose. The inhibitory properties of these agents are greatest for *glucoamylase,* followed by sucrose, maltose and dextrose respectively. Examples of α-glucosidase inhibitors are Acarbose, Miglitol and Voglibose

A. Acarbose (Diabose, Acboz)

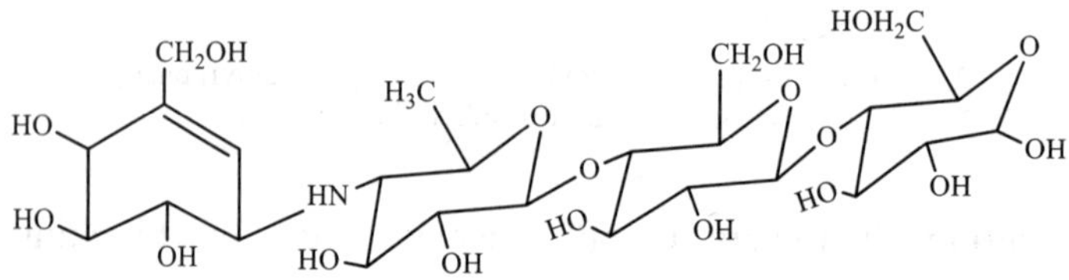

It is a pseudo tetra saccharide containing an unsaturated cyclitol moiety

Mechanism of action: It act as an oral hypoglycemic agent by inhibiting *α-glucosidase* and reduces sugar absorption in the gastro-intestinal tract (GIT).

Use: It is used as antidiabetic agent.

B.Voglibose (Volix, Vocarb)

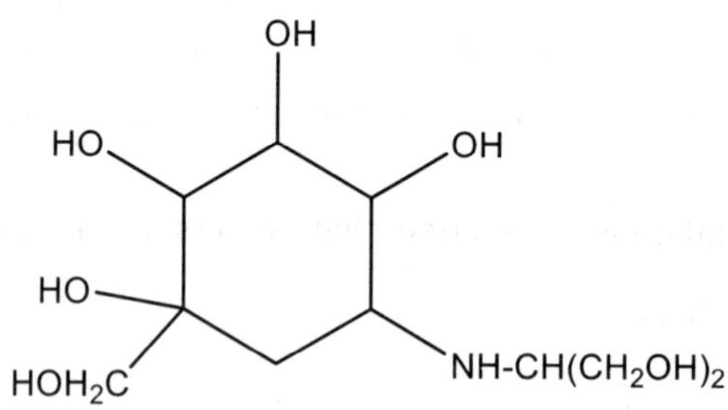

5 - [(1,3 - Dihydroxy propan - 2 - yl) amino] - 1 - (hydroxy methyl) cyclohexane - 1, 2, 3, 4 - tetrol

Mechanism of action: It acts as an oral hypoglycemic agent by inhibiting *α-glucosidase* and reduces sugar absorption in the gastro-intestinal tract (GIT).

Use: It is used as antidiabetic agent.

Chapter

LOCAL ANAESTHETICS

13

1. INTRODUCTION

Local anaesthetics are agents, that when administered locally, produces reversible loss of sensation in local areas of the body. They interrupt pain impulses in a specific region of the body without loss of patient consciousness. They are widely used in dentistry, in ophthalmology, in minor surgical operations including endoscopy and in relieving pain in certain medical conditions like tumors growing in the spine. Local anesthetics are also applied topically for the temporary relief of pain from insect bite, burns and other surface of wounds.

1.1 Mechanism of Action

Local anesthetics produces anaesthesia by inhibiting excitation of nerve endings or by blocking conduction in peripheral nerves. The nerve fiber is cylindrical in shape and surrounded by a semi-permeable membrane. This membrane is made up of protein and lipids. Some proteins act as channel or pore for the passage of sodium and potassium ion through the membrane. The movement of nerve impulse, along with a nerve fiber associated with a change in the permeability of the membrane. In neuron, excitable membrane have more Na^+ ion outside in resting state and K^+ ion inside.

When impulse conduction take place the pores widen and sodium ions (Na^+) move inside the fiber. At the same time, potassium ion (K^+) diffuses out through other pores. The entire process is called "depolarization". Immediately after the nerve impulse had passed, the pores again become smaller. Sodium ions are pumped out of the fiber at the same time potassium ions are transported into the fiber. The ability of local anaesthetic to bind to sodium channel is known as "State dependent block". It binds to sodium channel during depolarization (when open and activated). Local anaesthetics reversibly bind to these Na^+ channels and thereby inhibit the excitation of nerve endings and thus produces anaesthesia.

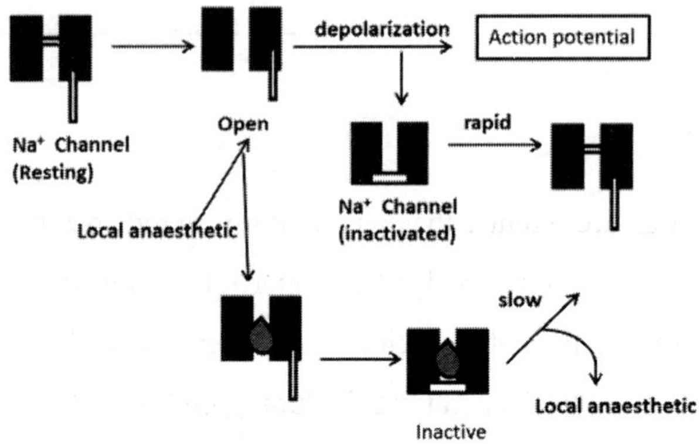

Fig. 13.1 Depolarization of Voltage Gated Na^+ Channel

1.2 Structure Activity Relationship

Most of the local anesthetic consists of three parts namely lipophilic center, intermediate alkyl chain and hydrophilic centre. The intermediate alkyl chain is either ester or amides. (Fig.13.2)

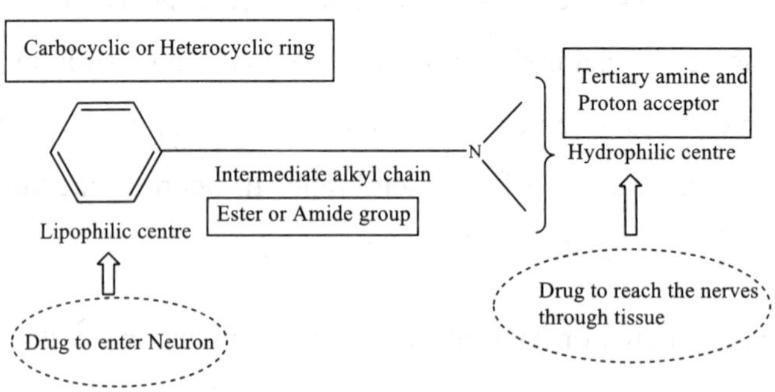

Fig. 13.2 Common Structural Features of Local Anaesthetics

- **Lipophilic center** which is responsible for lipid solubility is essential for local anesthetic activity.
- Lipid solubility plays an important role in the action of local anaesthetics, since their action depends on their ability to penetrate the cell membrane of the axon.

- Lipophilic center is either a carbocyclic ring or heterocyclic ring system.
- The **hydrophilic center** is an essential factor in transporting the drug to the membrane, to the cell and to the receptor.
- The hydrophilic group can be in the form of a secondary or tertiary amine or part of a nitrogen heterocycle. Tertiary amines are less irritant to tissue so it is more useful.
- Most clinically useful local anesthetics have a tertiary alkyl amine which readily forms water soluble salts suitable for pharmaceutical preparations.
- The presence of piperidino and pyrrolidino group as hydrophilic center gives rise to almost identical activity.
- The best local anesthetic action is obtained when the lipophilic and hydrophilic center are in balance. The partition coefficient of local anesthetic drug having identical structure increases the activity to a maximum. Once the peak is reached the activity starts decreasing though the partition-coefficient enhances.
- The pKa value of local anesthetic lies between 7.5 to 9.5. The compounds with pKa value below 7.5 are not sufficiently ionized at physiological pH to be effective in bringing anaesthesia. The drug with pKa value above 9.5 is almost fully ionized they are less effective, because it cannot penetrate the cell membrane.
- Mostly local anesthetics are available as salt form which increases the stability and solubility.
- **Linkage** between the aromatic ring and the amino group is either ester or amide. They may be either short hydrocarbon chain or oxygen, nitrogen or sulfur atoms.
- Ester type local anaesthetics are easily metabolized and have shorter duration of action. Due to slow metabolism, amide type local anaesthetics have longer duration of action.

- A study of homologous series formed by substituting the aryl ring of local anesthetic by alkyl, alkoxy and alkyl amino group, showed that, the partition coefficient of member of series increases with increase in the numbers of methylene group in the substituent of the series. In general, maximum activity is achieved for the C_4 to C_6 homologue. Similarly, substitution of the hydrophilic center showed that, as the number of carbon atom increases the partition coefficient as well as activity increases.
- Local anaesthetics bind to plasma and tissue protein by three forces Vander - Waal's force, Dipole-Dipole attraction and Electrostatic Forces.

2. CLASSIFICATION

Based on chemical structure local anaesthetic can be classified as

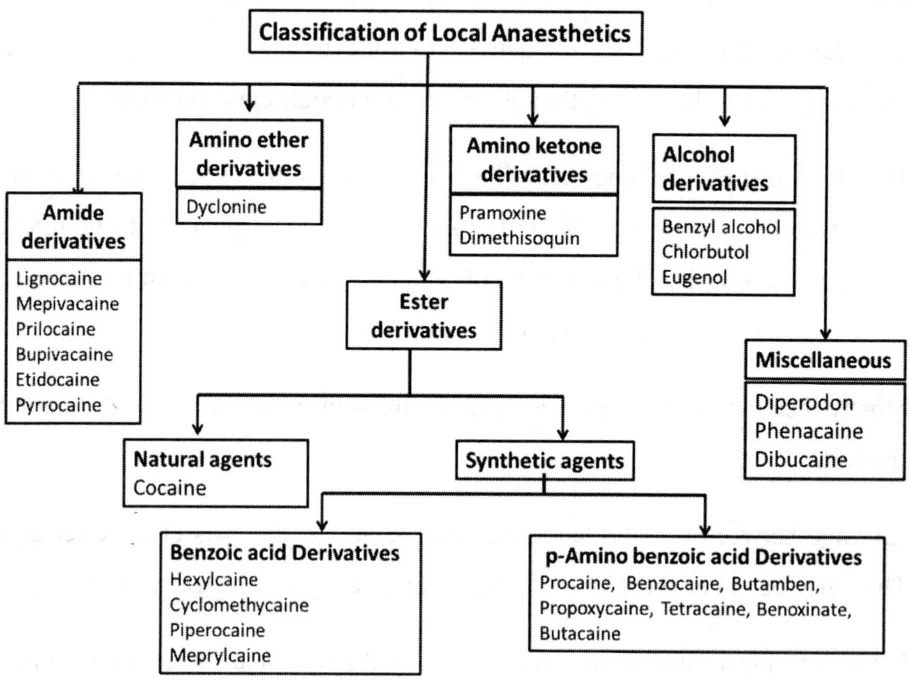

2.1 Ester Based

Cocaine was the first anaesthetic to be discovered and is only naturally occurring anesthetic. In 1884, it was used in patients with glaucoma. Procaine was the first synthetic local anaesthetic.

Ester type of local anaesthetics has

- ✓ Shorter duration of action and less intense analgesia
- ✓ Causes allergic reaction
- ✓ Metabolized in plasma by *Pseudo choline esterase*
- ✓ Unstable in solution.

2.1.1 Natural Agents

A. Cocaine (Goprelto)

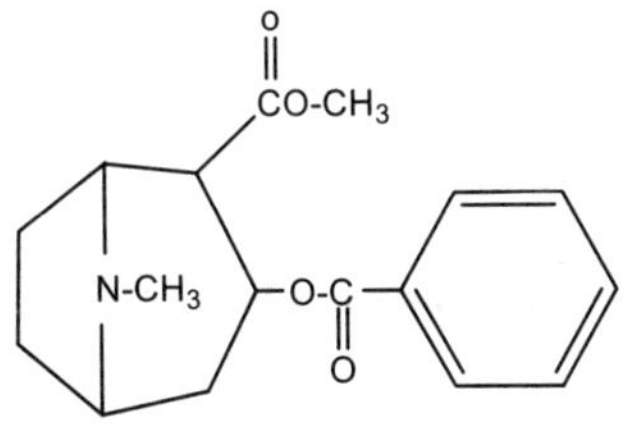

Methyl - 3 - (benzoyloxy) - 8 - methyl - 8 - azabicyclo [3.2.1] octane - 2 - carboxylate

It is a tropane alkaloid obtained from the leaves of *Erythroxylon cocoa*. It is a drug of abuse and causes addiction after prolong use. It was discovered in 1860 and used till 1884. Later on, due to its addictive potential, it is labeled as drug of abuse and discontinued.

Mechanism of action: It is a central nervous systems (CNS) stimulant and local anesthetic. The mechanism of action of cocaine as local anesthetic is by blocking the voltage gated sodium channels in the neuronal cell membrane. By stabilizing neuronal membranes, cocaine inhibits the initiation and conduction of nerve impulses and produces a reversible loss of sensation. Cocaine binds to the dopamine, serotonin and nor-epinephrine transport proteins and inhibits the re-uptake of dopamine, serotonin and nor-epinephrine into pre-synaptic neurons. This leads to an accumulation of the respective neurotransmitters in the synaptic cleft and is most responsible for the addictive property of cocaine. Cocaine also shows vasoconstrictive properties due its blockade of nor-epinephrine reuptake in the autonomic nervous system

Use: It is applied topically as a 2% solution for anaesthesia of the ear, nose, throat, upper respiratory tract, rectum and vagina.

2.1.2 Synthetic Agents

2.1.2.1 Derivatives of Benzoic Acid

A. Hexylcaine (Cycaine)

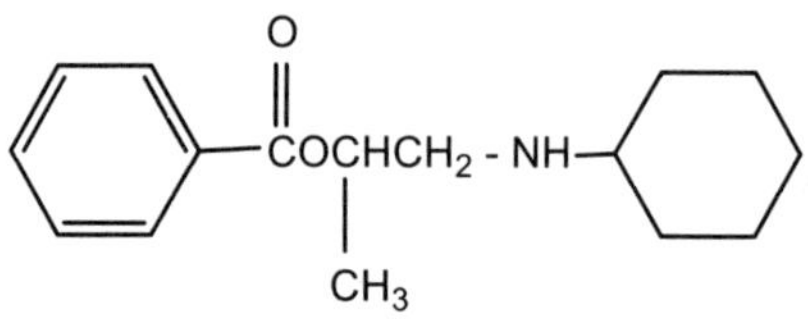

1 - Cyclohexylamino- propan-2-yl benzoate

It is also known as Osmocaine

Mechanism of action: Local anesthetic activity is by blocking the voltage gated sodium channels in the neuronal cell membrane. By stabilizing neuronal membranes, it inhibits the initiation and conduction of nerve impulses and produces a reversible loss of sensation.

Use: It is used as surface anaesthesia.

B. Cyclomethylcaine (Surfcaine)

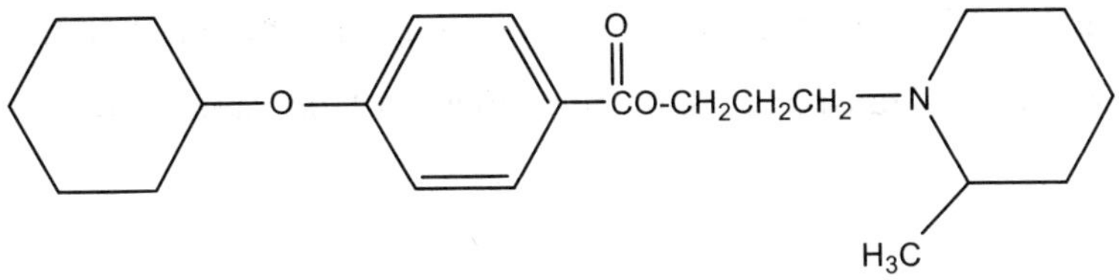

3 - (2 - Methyl piperidino) propyl - 4 - (cyclo hexyloxy) benzoate

Mechanism of action: Local anesthetic activity is by blocking the voltage gated sodium channels in the neuronal cell membrane. By stabilizing neuronal membranes, it inhibits the initiation and conduction of nerve impulses and produces a reversible loss of sensation.

Use: It is used to relieve pain from damaged skin, mucous membrane of rectum, vagina and urinary bladder.

C. Piperocaine (Metycaine)

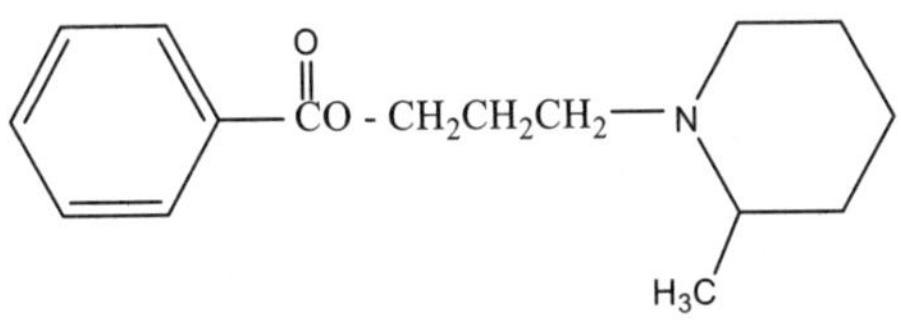

3 - (2 - Methyl piperidino) propyl benzoate

Mechanism of action: Local anesthetic activity is by blocking the voltage gated sodium channels in the neuronal cell membrane. By stabilizing neuronal membranes, it inhibits the initiation and conduction of nerve impulses and produces a reversible loss of sensation.

Use: It is used for eye, throat and caudal analgesia.

D. Meprylcaine (Epirocaine, Oracaine)

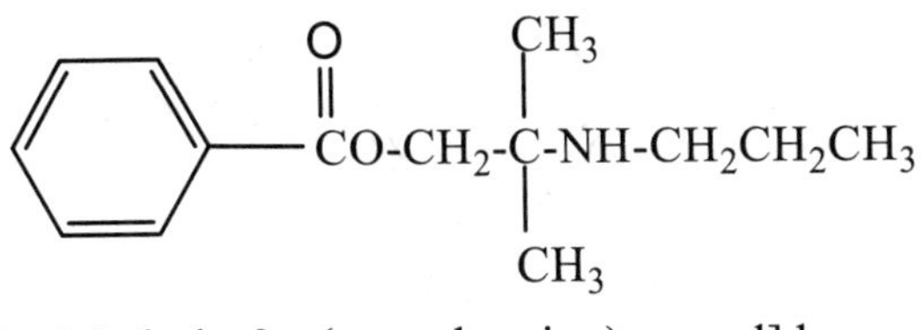

[2 - Methyl - 2 - (propyl amino) propyl] benzoate

It is a local anesthetic with stimulant activity

Mechanism of action: It acts as local anesthetic through inhibition of sodium channels. It also inhibits monoamine transporter and the reuptake of dopamine, nor-epinephrine and serotonin.

Use: It is used as local anesthetic.

2.1.2.2 Derivatives of p-Amino Benzoic Acid

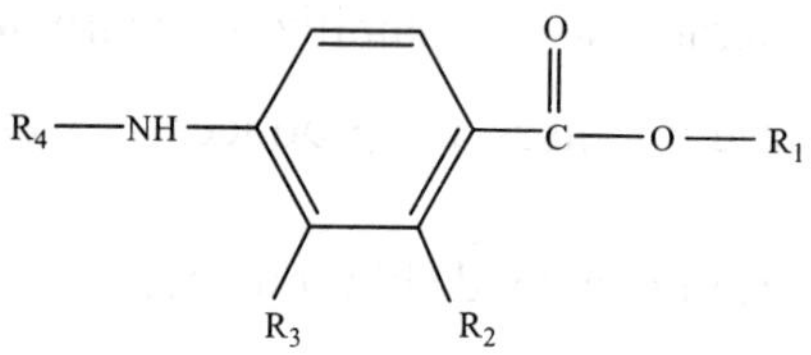

S. No	Name	R_1	R_2	R_3	R_4
1.	Benzocaine	$- C_2H_5$	-H	-H	-H
2.	Butamben	$- CH_2CH_2CH_2CH_3$	-H	-H	-H
3.	Procaine	$- CH_2CH_2 - N - (C_2H_5)_2$	-H	-H	-H
4.	Butacaine	$- CH_2CH_2CH_2 - N - (C_4H_9)_2$	-H	-H	-H
5.	Propoxycaine	$- CH_2CH_2 - N - (C_2H_5)_2$	$- OCH_2CH_2CH_3$	-H	-H
6.	Tetracaine	$- CH_2CH_2 - N - (CH_3)_2$	-H	-H	$-C_4H_9$
7.	Benoxinate	$- CH_2CH_2 - N - (C_2H_5)_2$	-H	$-O(CH_2)_3 CH_3$	-H

A. Benzocaine (Anaesthesin)

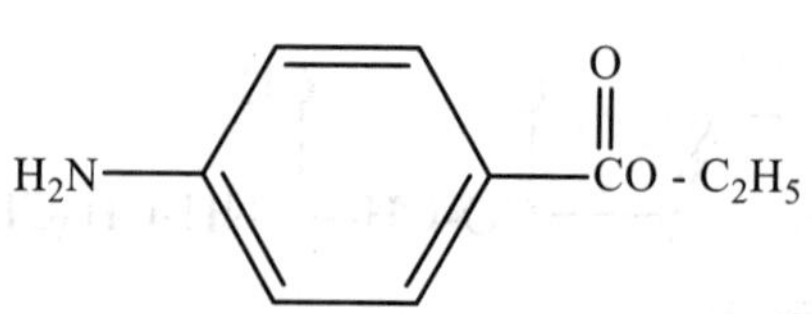

Ethyl - p - amino benzoate

Synthesis

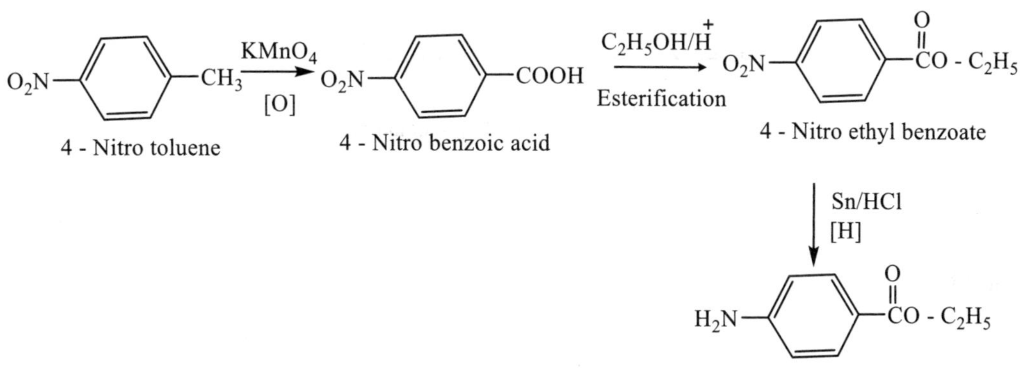

Benzocanie

Mechanism of action: Local anesthetic activity is by blocking the voltage gated sodium channels in the neuronal cell membrane. By stabilizing neuronal membranes, it inhibits the initiation and conduction of nerve impulses and produces a reversible loss of sensation.

Use: Being insoluble in nature, it is generally used as topical anaesthesia to get rid of the pain caused by wounds, ulcers and mucous surface.

B. Butamben (Catecaine)

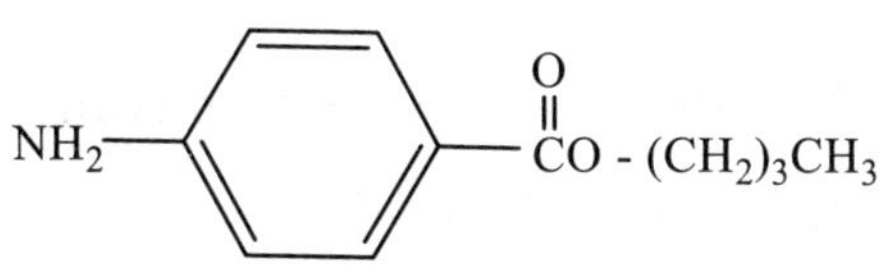

Butyl - p - amino benzoate

Mechanism of action: Local anesthetic activity is by blocking the voltage gated sodium channels in the neuronal cell membrane. By stabilizing neuronal membranes, it inhibits the initiation and conduction of nerve impulses and produces a reversible loss of sensation.

Use: It is used as topical anaesthetics to get rid of the pain caused by wounds, ulcers and mucous surface. Because of its low solubility, it is more efficacious than Benzocaine.

C. Procaine (Novocaine)

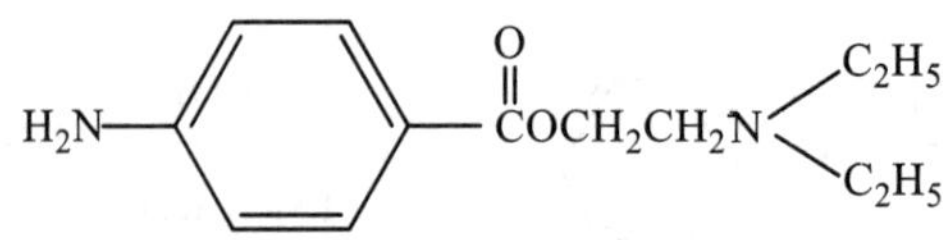

2 - (Diethyl amino) ethyl - p - amino benzoate

Synthesis

Method I:

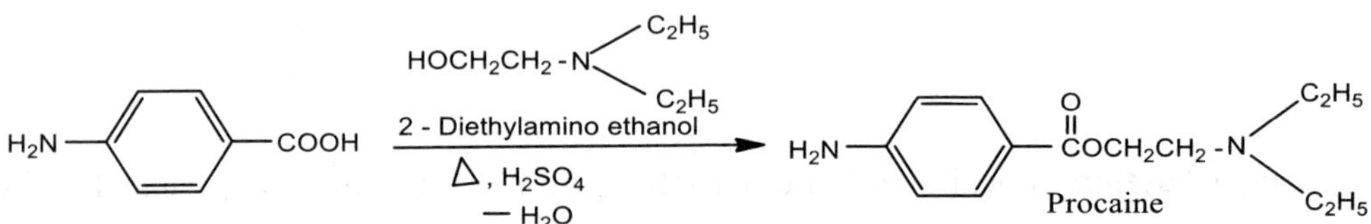

4 - Amino benzoic acid

Method II:

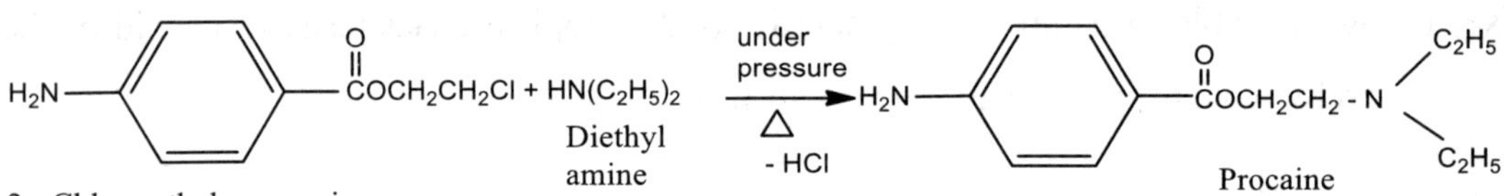

2 - Chloro ethyl - p - amino benzoate

Mechanism of action: Local anesthetic activity is by blocking the voltage gated sodium channels in the neuronal cell membrane. By stabilizing neuronal membranes, it inhibits the initiation and conduction of nerve impulses and produces a reversible loss of sensation.

Use: It is less toxic and most commonly used local anaesthetics.

D. Butacaine (Butyn)

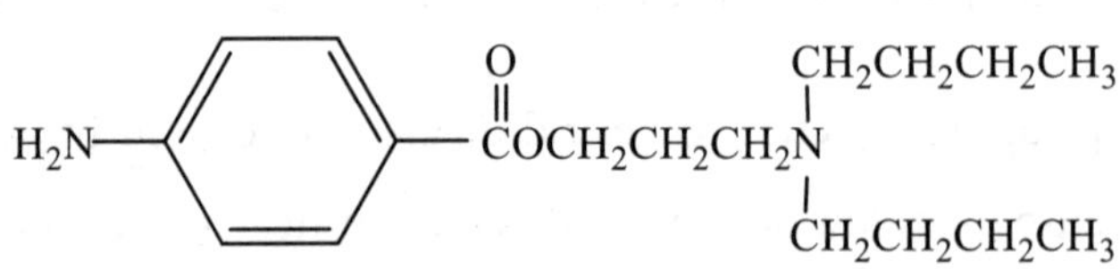

3 - (Dibutyl amino) propyl - 4 - amino benzoate

Mechanism of action: Local anesthetic activity is by blocking the voltage gated sodium channels in the neuronal cell membrane. By stabilizing neuronal membranes, it inhibits the initiation and conduction of nerve impulses and produces a reversible loss of sensation.

Use: It is used as local anaesthetics.

E.Propoxycaine (Blockain)

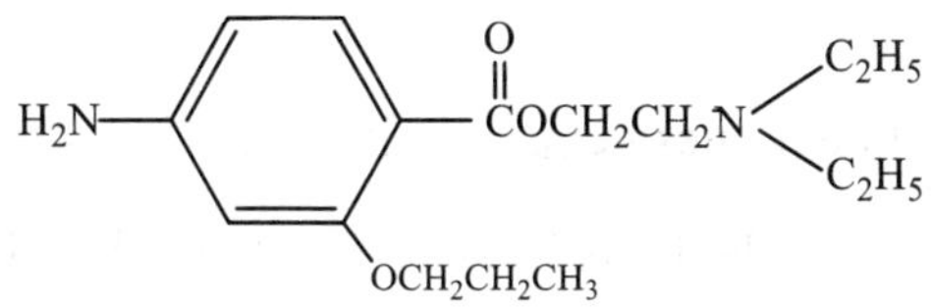

2 - (Diethyl amino) ethyl - 4 - amino - 2 - propoxy benzoate

It is a local anesthetic of the ester type that has a rapid onset of action and a longer duration of action than procaine.

Mechanism of action: Local anesthetic activity is by blocking the voltage gated sodium channels in the neuronal cell membrane. By stabilizing neuronal membranes, it inhibits the initiation and conduction of nerve impulses and produces a reversible loss of sensation.

Use: It is used as local anaesthetics.

F. Tetracaine (Amethocaine)

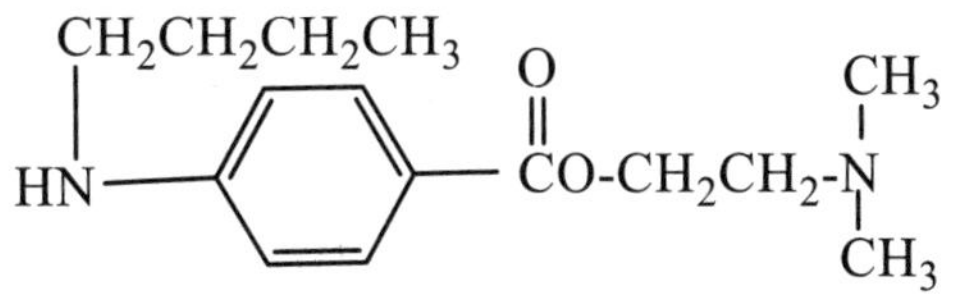

2 - (Dimethyl amino) - ethyl - 4 - (butyl amino) benzoate

Mechanism of action: Local anesthetic activity is by blocking the voltage gated sodium channels in the neuronal cell membrane. By stabilizing neuronal membranes, it inhibits the initiation and conduction of nerve impulses and produces a reversible loss of sensation.

Use: It is used in surface infiltration and spinal anaesthesia.

G. Benoxinate (Oxybuprocaine or BNX)

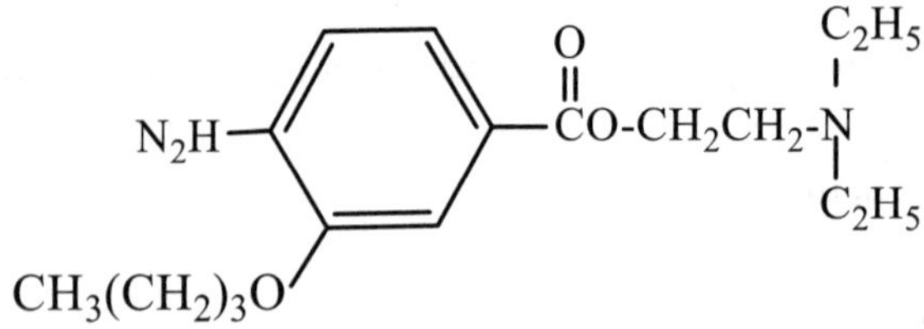

2 - Diethylamino ethyl - 4 - amino - 3 - butoxy benzoate

Mechanism of action: Local anesthetic activity is by blocking the voltage gated sodium channels in the neuronal cell membrane. By stabilizing neuronal membranes, it inhibits the initiation and conduction of nerve impulses and produces a reversible loss of sensation.

Use: It is a local anesthetic, used especially in ophthalmology and otolaryngology.

2.2 Amide Based

Amide based local anaesthetics have longer duration of action, more intense analgesics. It metabolizes in liver and very stable in solution.

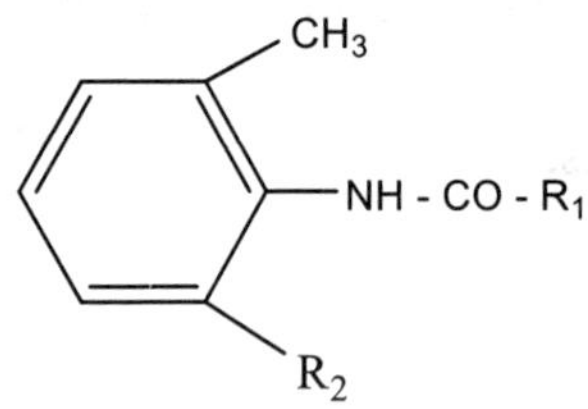

S.No.	Name	R_1	R_2
1.	Lignocaine	$- CH_2 - N - (C_2H_5)_2$	$- CH_3$
2.	Mepivacaine	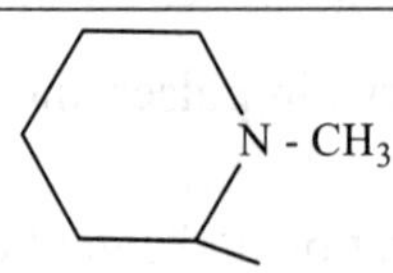	$- CH_3$

3.	Prilocaine	$-CH(CH_3)-NH-(CH_2)_2CH_3$	- H
4.	Etidocaine	$-CH(CH_2CH_3)-N(C_2H_5)(CH_2CH_2CH_3)$	- CH_3

A. Lignocaine (Xylocaine)

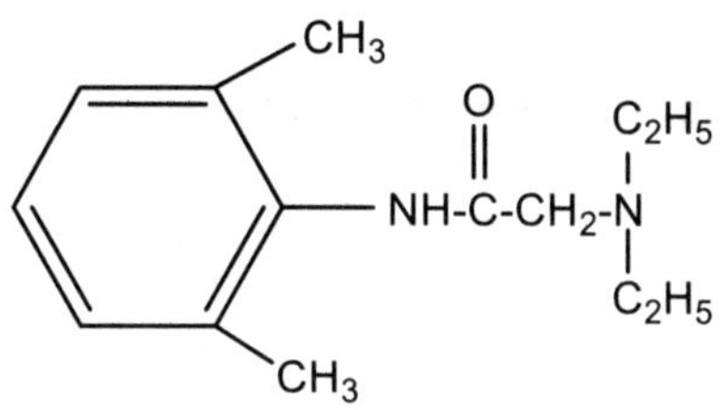

N,N - (Diethyl amino aceto) - 2, 6 - xylidine

It is also known as Lidocaine, which is a synthetic amino ethyl amide with local anesthetic and antiarrhythmic properties.

Mechanism of action: Local anesthetic activity is by blocking the voltage gated sodium channels in the neuronal cell membrane. By stabilizing neuronal membranes, it inhibits the initiation and conduction of nerve impulses and produces a reversible loss of sensation. Blocking sodium channels in the conduction system, as well as the muscle cells of the heart, it acts as antiarrhythmic.

Use: It is used for terminal infiltration, block, epidural and spinal anaesthesia during operational interventions in dentistry, otolaryngology, obstetrics and gynaecology. It has local vasodilation action but usually used with vasoconstrictor adrenaline, to prolong the local anesthetic activity.

B. Mepivacaine (Carbocaine)

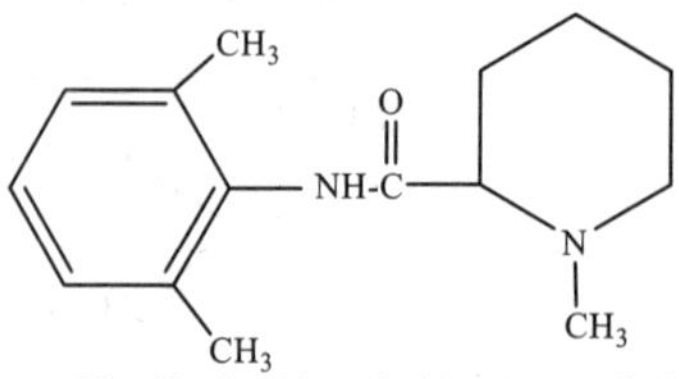

N - (2, 6 - Dimethyl) - 1 - methyl -
2 - piperidine carboxamide

Mechanism of action: Local anesthetic activity is by blocking the voltage gated sodium channels in the neuronal cell membrane. By stabilizing neuronal membranes, it inhibits the initiation and conduction of nerve impulses and produces a reversible loss of sensation.

Use: It is a local anesthetic agent most commonly used for regional or intrasynovial analgesia of the foot.

C. Etidocaine (Duranest)

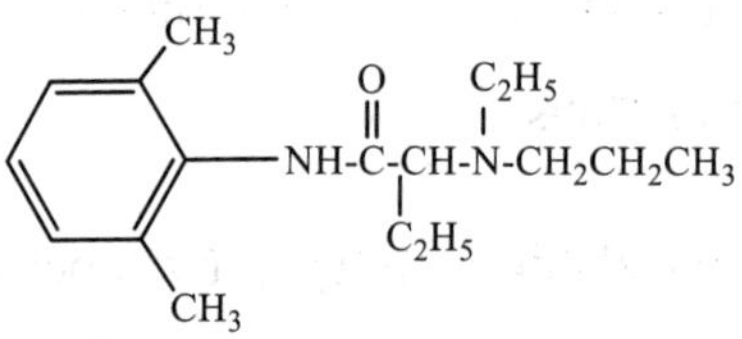

N - (2, 6 - Dimethyl phenyl) - 2 - (ethyl
(propyl) amino) butanamide

Mechanism of action: Local anesthetic activity is by blocking the voltage gated sodium channels in the neuronal cell membrane. By stabilizing neuronal membranes, it inhibits the initiation and conduction of nerve impulses and produces a reversible loss of sensation.

Use: It is used as anesthetic drug during surgical procedures and labor and delivery.

D. Prilocaine (Citanest)

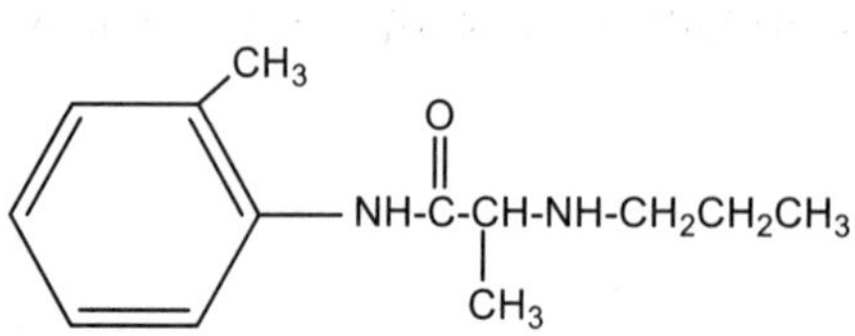

N - (2 - Methyl phenyl) - 2 - (propyl
amino) propanamide

Mechanism of action: Local anesthetic activity is by blocking the voltage gated sodium channels in the neuronal cell membrane. By stabilizing neuronal membranes, it inhibits the initiation and conduction of nerve impulses and produces a reversible loss of sensation.

Use: It has low cardiac toxicity it is commonly used for intravenous regional anaesthesia.

2.3 Miscellaneous

A. Phenacaine (Tropex)

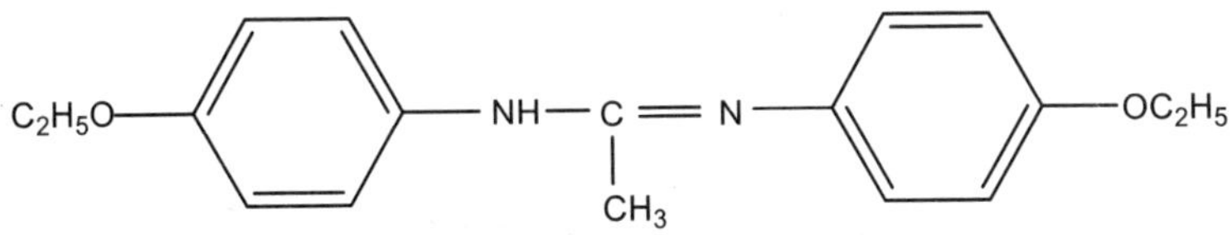

N,N' - bis (4 - ethoxy phenyl) ethanimidamide

Mechanism of action: Local anesthetic activity is by blocking the voltage gated sodium channels in the neuronal cell membrane. By stabilizing neuronal membranes, it inhibits the initiation and conduction of nerve impulses and produces a reversible loss of sensation.

Use: It is used as 1% solution mainly for producing local anaesthesia of eye.

B. Diperodon

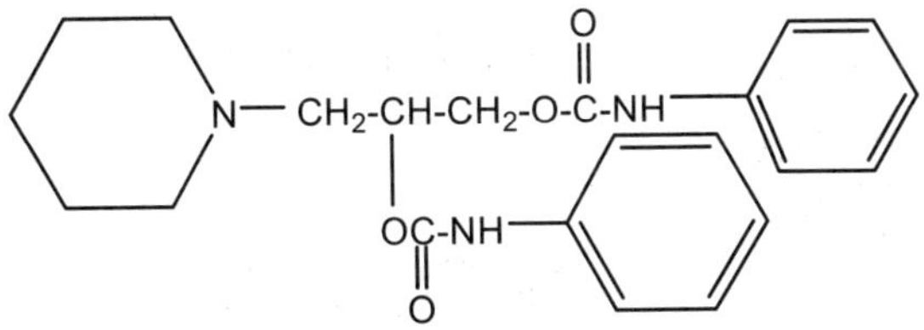

3 - (1 - Piperidinyl) - bis (phenyl carbamate) - 1,2 - propanediol

Mechanism of action: Local anesthetic activity is by blocking the voltage gated sodium channels in the neuronal cell membrane. By stabilizing neuronal membranes, it inhibits the initiation and conduction of nerve impulses and produces a reversible loss of sensation.

Use: It is a potent surface anesthetic applied to the skin for abrasions, pruritus and irritations.

C. Dibucaine (Cinchocaine)

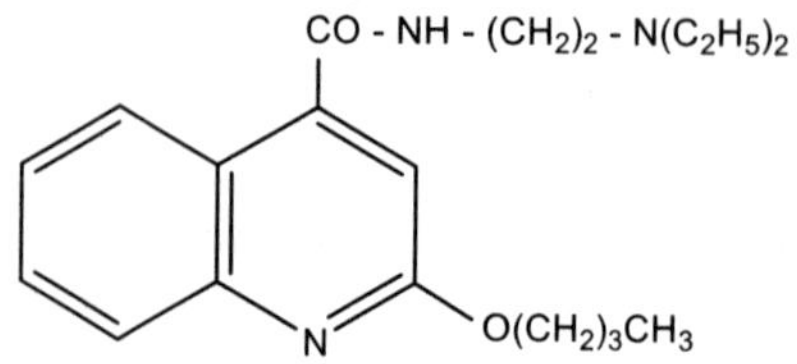

2 - Butoxy - N - [2 - (diethyl amino) ethy] - 4 - quinoline carboxamide

Synthesis

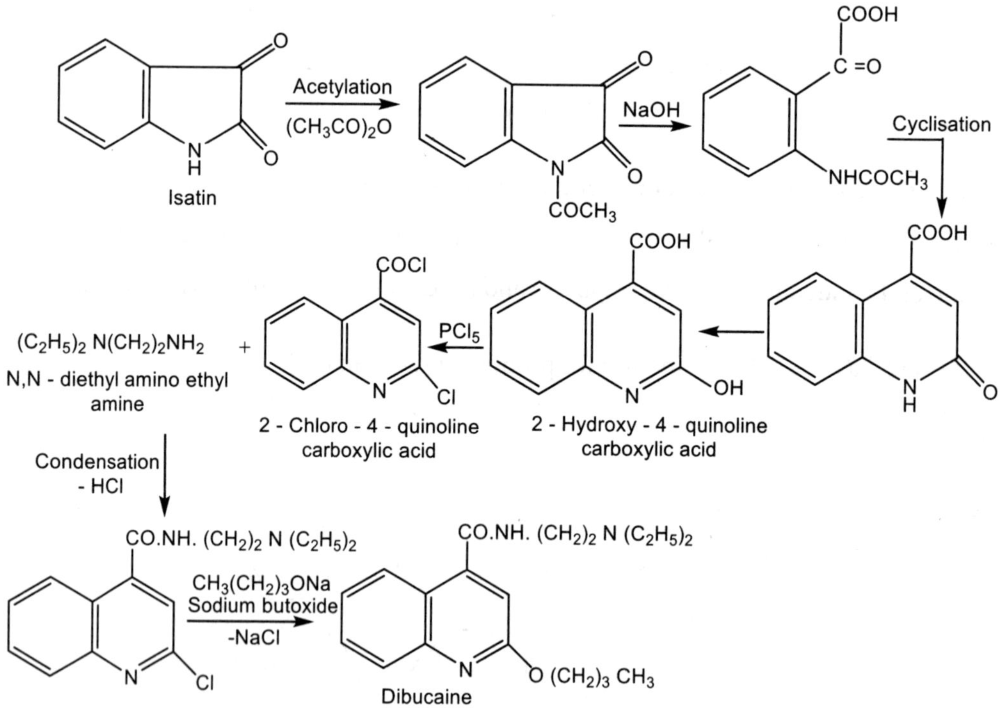

Mechanism of action: Local anesthetic activity is by blocking the voltage gated sodium channels in the neuronal cell membrane. By stabilizing neuronal membranes, it inhibits the initiation and conduction of nerve impulses and produces a reversible loss of sensation.

Use: It is one of the most potent and long acting local anaesthetics used as infiltration, surface and spinal anaesthesia.

Index

A

Acarbose, 160, **166**
Acetazolamide, 62, 4**2**
Acetomenaphthone, 105, **106**
Amiloride, 62, **72**
Amiodarone, 91, **98**
Amlodipine, 50, 55, **56**
Amyl nitrate, 50, **51**
Anisindione, 108, **109**
Astemizole, 8, **22**
Azatadine maleate, 8, **19**
Azathioprine, 29, **40**

B

Benazepril hydrochloride, 76, **90**
Benoxinate, 170, 174, **178**
Benzocaine, 170, 1**74**
Bepridil hydrochloride, 50, **59**
Betamethasone, 144, **146**
Bleomycin, 29, **44**
Bosentan, 113, **120**
Buclizine hydrochloride, 8, 13, **14**
Bumetanide, 62, **70**
Busulfan, 29, **34**
Butacaine, 170, 174, **176**
Butamben, 170, 174, **175**

C

Captopril, 77, **87**
Cetirizine, 8, **21**
Chlorambucil, 29, **34**
Chlorcyclizine hydrochloride, 8, 12, **13**
Chlorothiazide, 62, 67, **68**
Chlorpheniramine maleate, 8, **15**
Chlorpropamide, 160, **162**
Cholestyramine, 100, **103**
Cholestipol, 100, **104**
Cimetidine, 8, **24**
Cisplatin, 29, **49**
Clemastine fumarate, 8, **10**
Clofibrate, 100, **102**
Clonidine hydrochloride, 76, **80**
Clopidogrel, **110**
Cocaine, 170, **171**
Cortisone, 144, **145**
Cromolyn sodium, **4**
Cyclomethycaine, 170, **173**
Cyclophosphamide, 29, **33**
Cyclothiazide, 62, 67, **69**
Cyproheptadine hydrochloride, 8, **19**
Cytarabine, 29, **38**

D

Dactinomycin, 29, **45**
Daunorubicin, 29, **44**
Dexamethasone, 144, **147**
Diazoxide, 76, **84**
Dibucaine, 170, **182**
Dichlorphenamide, 62, **66**
Diethylstilbestrol, **137**
Digitoxin, 113, 117, **118**
Digoxin, 113, 117, **118**
Diltiazem hydrochloride, 50, **58**
Dimenhydrinate, 8, **9**
Diperadon, 170, **181**
Diphenhydramine hydrochloride, 8, **9**
Diphenylpyraline hydrochloride, 8, **11**
Dipyridamole, 50, **59**
Disopyramide phosphate, 91, **93**
Doxorubicin, 29, **44**
Doxylamine succinate, 8, **10**

E

Enalapril, 77, 87, **88**
Ethacrynic acid, 62, **71**
Etidocaine, 170, 179, **180**
Etoposide, 29, **47**

F

Famotidine, 8, **25**
Felodipine, 50, 55, **57**
Floxuridine, 29, **37**
Fluorouracil, 29, **36**
Furosemide, 62, **70**

G

Glimepiride, 160, **162**
Glipizide, 160, **162**
Guanabenz acetate, 76, **82**
Guanethidine monosulphate, 76, **79**

H

Hexylcaine, 170, **172**
Hydralazine hydrochloride, 76, **83**
Hydrochlorthiazide, 62, 67, **68**
Hydrocortisone, 144, **145**
Hydroflumethiazide, 62, 67, **69**

I

Insulin, 153
Isosorbide dinitrite, 50, **52**

L

Lansoprazole, 8, **27**
Levocetirizine, 8, **21**
Levonorgestrel, 140-41, **142,** 143
Lidocaine hydrochloride, 91, **94**
Lignocaine, 170, 178, **179**
Lisinopril, 76, 88, **89**
Loratadine, 8, **22**
Lorcainide hydrochloride, 91, **97**
Lovastatin, 100, **101**
L-Thyronine, **151**
L-Thyroxine, **151**

M

Mannitol, 62, **73**
Meandione, 105, **106**
Mechlorethamine, 29, **31**
Meclizine hydrochloride, 8, 12, **13**
Melphalan, 29, **34**
Mepivacaine, 170, 178, **180**
Meprylcaine, 170, **173**
Mercaptopurine, 29, **39**
Metformin, 160, **163**
Methazolamide, 62, **65**
Methimazole, 152, **153**
Methotrexate, 29, **41**
Methyldopate hydrochloride, 76, **81**
Mexiletine hydrochloride, 91, **96**
Mifepristone, **141**
Minoxidil, 76, **84**
Mitotane, 29, **48**

N

Nandralone, **133**
Nateglinide, 160, **165**
Nesiritide, 113, **119**
Nicardipine, 50, 55, **57**
Nifedipine, 50, 55, **56**
Nimodipine, 50, 55, **56**
Nitroglycerin, 50, **52**
Norgestrel, 140-41, **142,** 143

O

Oestradiol, 124, 130, **136**, 137, 142-4
Oestriol, **136**
Oestrone, 130, **136,** 137
Omeprazole, 8, **26**

P

Pantoprazole, 8, **27**
Pentaerythritol tetranitrate, 50, **52**
Phenacaine, 170, **181**
Phenindamine tartrate, 8, **17**
Phenytoin sodium, 91, **95**
Pioglitazone, 160, **164**
Piperocaine, 170, **173**
Prednisolone, 144, **146**
Prilocaine, 170, 179, **180**
Procainamide hydrochloride, 91, **93**
Procaine, 170, 174, **176**
Progesterone, 72, 124-25, 134, **135,** 140-43
Promethazine hydrochloride, 8, **18**
Propoxycaine, 170, 174, **177**
Propyl thiouracil, 152, **153**

Q

Quinapril hydrochloride, 76, 88, **89**
Quinidine sulphate, 91, **92**

R

Rabeprazole, 8, **27**
Ranitidine, 8, **25**
Repaglinide, 160, **165**
Reserpine, 76, **79**
Rosiglitazone, 160, **163**

S

Sildenafil, **138**
Sodium nitroprusside, 76, **85**
Sotalol, 91, **97**
Spironolactone, 62, **71**

T

Tadalafil, **139**
Testosterone, 124-25, 130-31, **132**, 133
Tetracaine, 170, 174, **177**
Tezosentan, 113, **121**
Thioguanine, 29, **40**
Thiotepa, 29, **35**
Timolol, 77, **78**
Tocainide hydrochloride, 91, **96**
Tolbutamide, 160, **161**
Triamterene, 62, **73**
Trimeprazine tartrate, 8, **18**
Tripelennamine hydrochloride, 8, **12**
Triprolidine hydrochloride, 8, **16**

V

Vearpamil, 50, **57**
Vinblastin sulphate, 29, **47**
Vincristin sulphate, 29, **47**
Voglibose, 160, **166**

W

Warfarin, **108**